Nutritious & Delicious

First published in 2022 by Dean Publishing
PO Box 119
Mt. Macedon, Victoria, 3441
Australia
deanpublishing.com

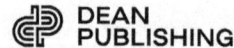

Copyright © Jady Roberts

Photography by Sarah Craven:
Food Stylist Photographer, sarahcravenphotography.com

All rights reserved. No part of this publication may be reproduced, stored in a retrieval system or transmitted in any way or by any means, electronic, mechanical, photocopying, recording or otherwise, without the prior written permission of the author.

Cataloguing-in-Publication Data
National Library of Australia
Title: Nutritious and Delicious
Edition: 1st edn
ISBN: 978-1-92545-245-7
Category: Cooking and Nutrition

This book is not intended as a substitute for nutritional or medical advice. The reader should regularly consult a physician or trained dietician in matters relating to their nutritional needs or general health. The ideas and recipes within this book are only the opinion of the author and are not intended to replace any medical or dietary advice or diagnose health issues or nutritional imbalances or needs.
The views and opinions expressed in this book are those of the author and do not necessarily reflect the official policy or position of any other agency, publisher, organization, employer or company. Assumptions made in the analysis are not reflective of the position of any entity other than the author(s)—and, these views are always subject to change, revision, and rethinking at any time. The author, publisher or organizations are not to be held responsible for misuse, reuse, recycled and cited and/or uncited copies of content within this book by others.

Nutritious & Delicious

Pure Wholesome Goodness

Jady Roberts

Check out the interactive book for pantry basics used in this book, as well as bonus recipes!

Light Lunches, Nourishing Bowls, Sharing Plates, Indulgences and more at **www.deanpublishing.com/nutritious**

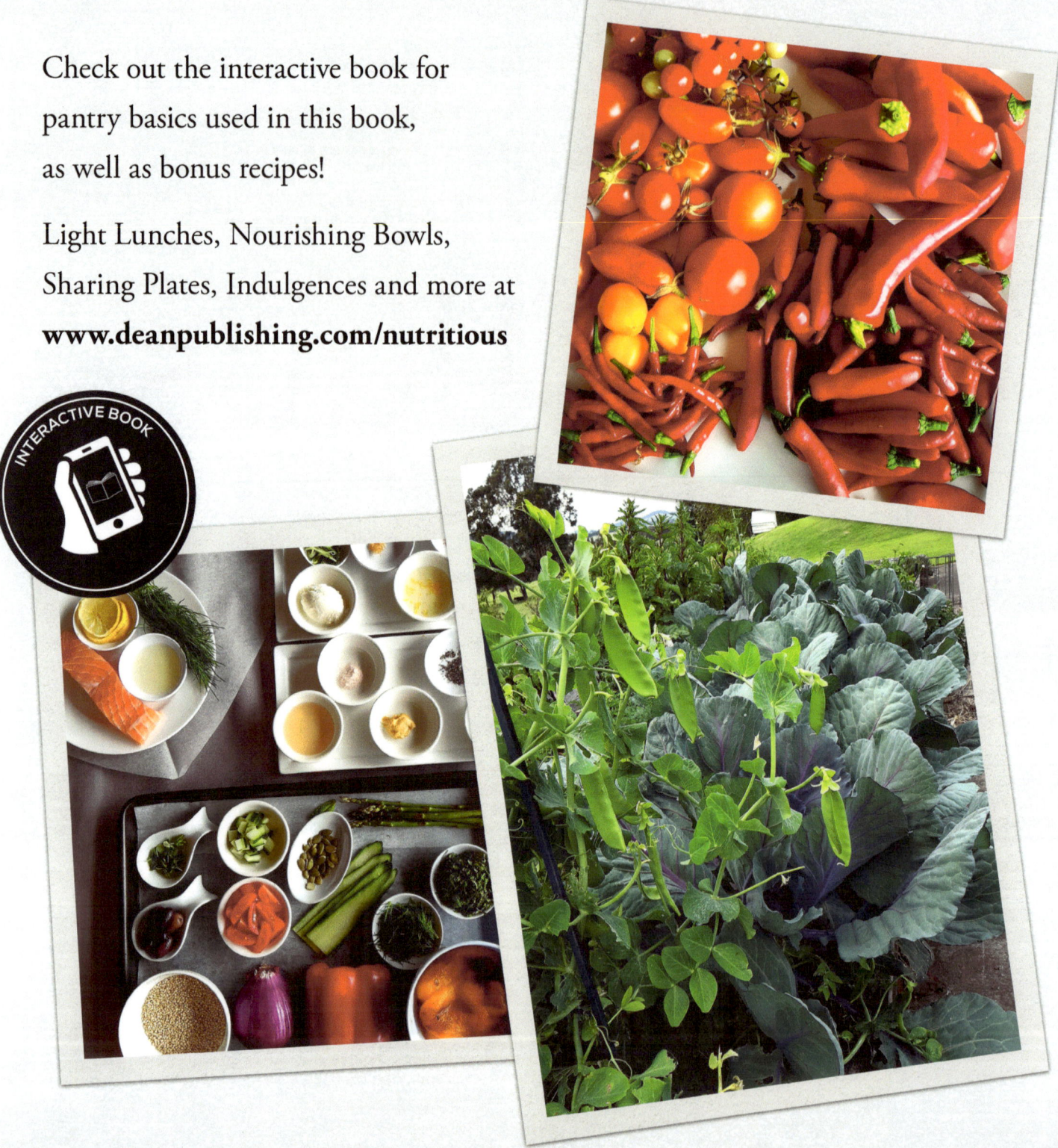

Contents

INTRODUCTION 9

FUNDAMENTALS OF NUTRITION 14

Carbohydrates	Herbs & Spices
Protein	Glycemic Index
Fats & Oils	Probiotics
Fibre	Planning Ahead
Vitamins & Minerals	Portion Control
Grains	

MORNING GLORY 36

STARTERS/LIGHT LUNCH 46

SHARING PLATES 56

NOURISHING BOWLS 64

THE MAIN EVENT 80

INDULGENCES 90

Combining wholesome foods in simple but mouthwatering recipes is my passion. Nutrition with flavour has never been so easy yet so exciting to achieve as you follow along with the definitions and recipes in my book that cover an array of salads, light meals, dinners, and desserts.

Best of all, you choose the level of cooking, from simple smoothies and fun healthy snacks right up to hosting a dinner party that is delightfully nutritious and beautiful for your guests, your culinary adventure starts here.

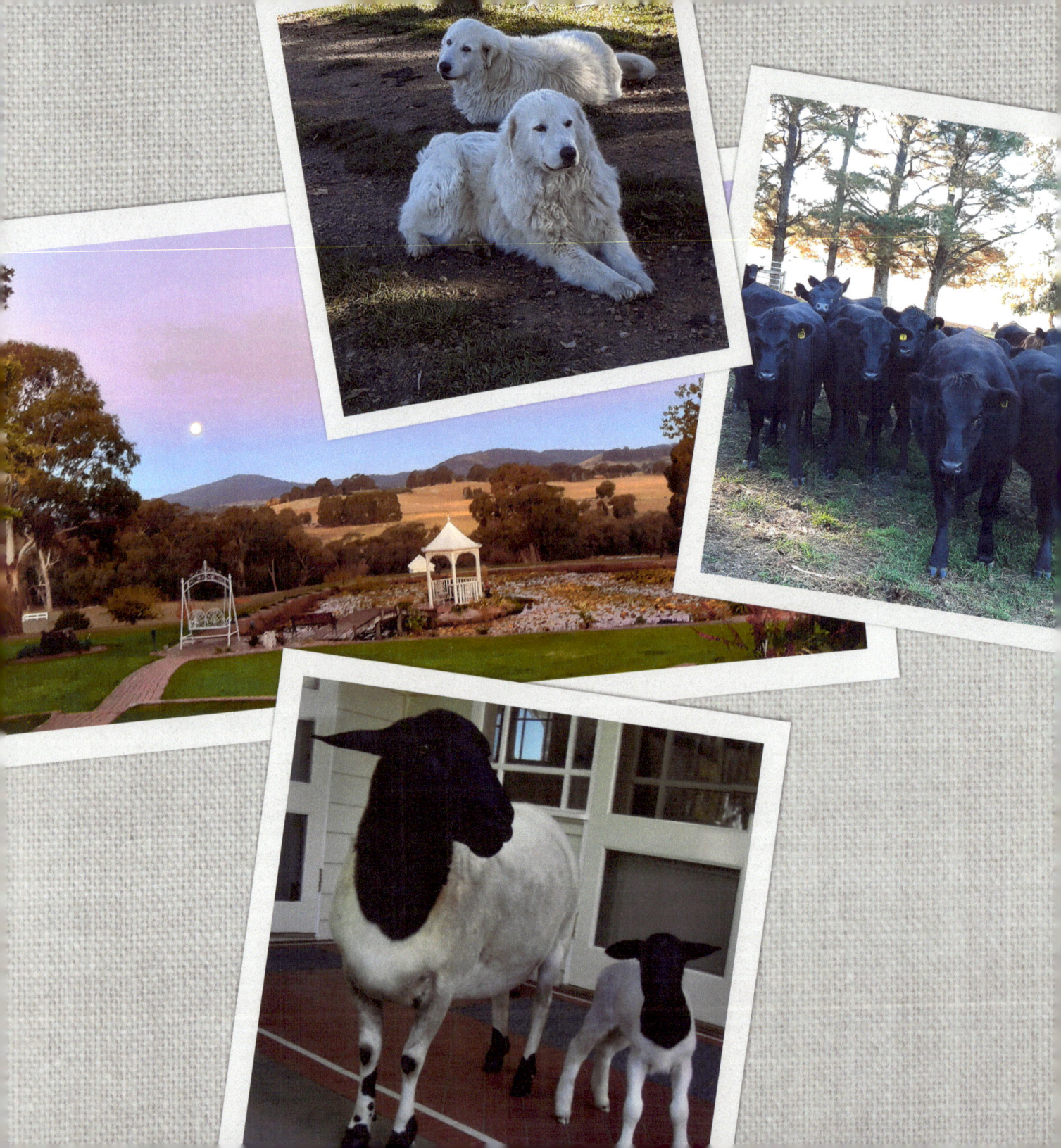

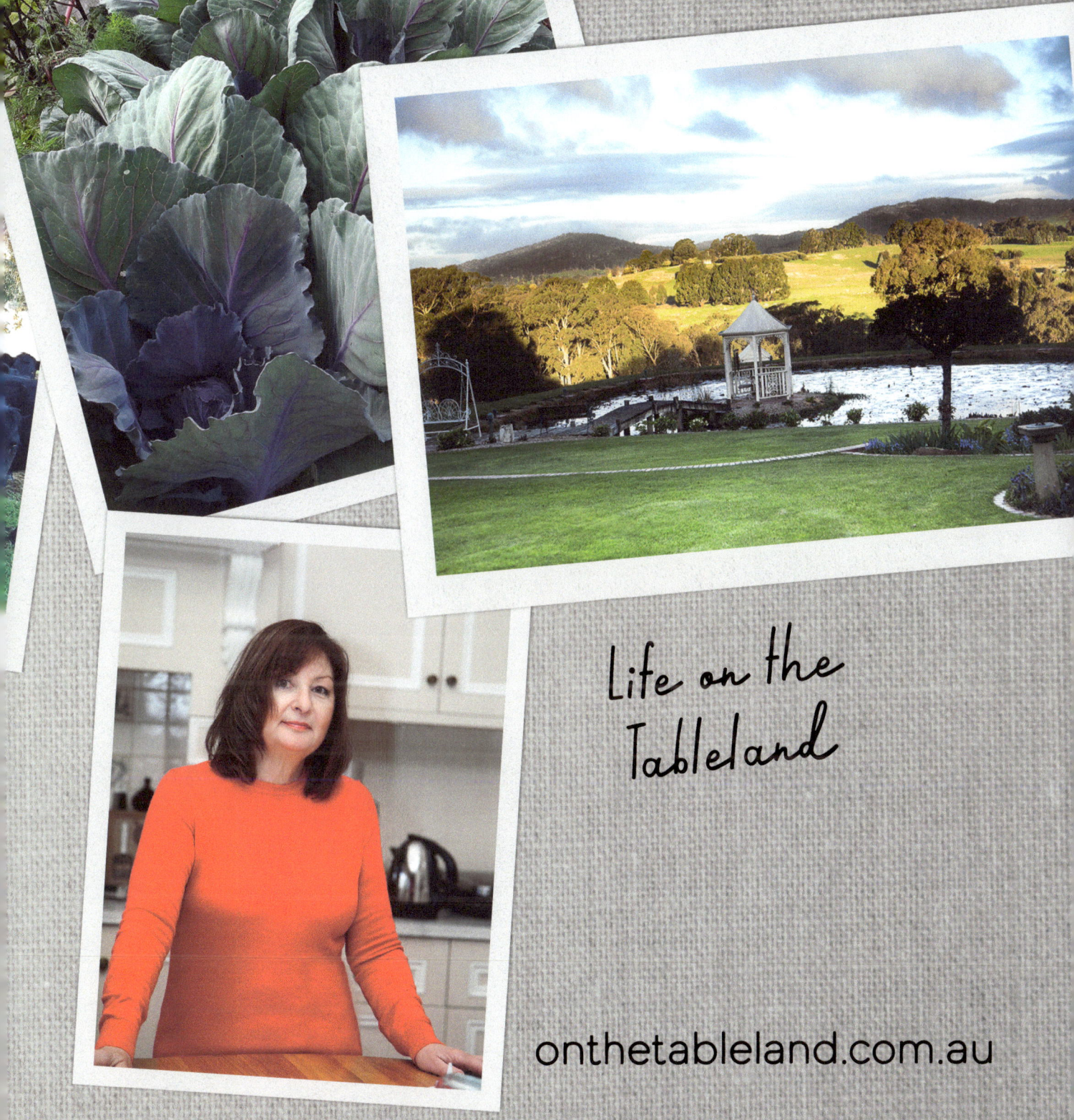

Life on the Tableland

onthetableland.com.au

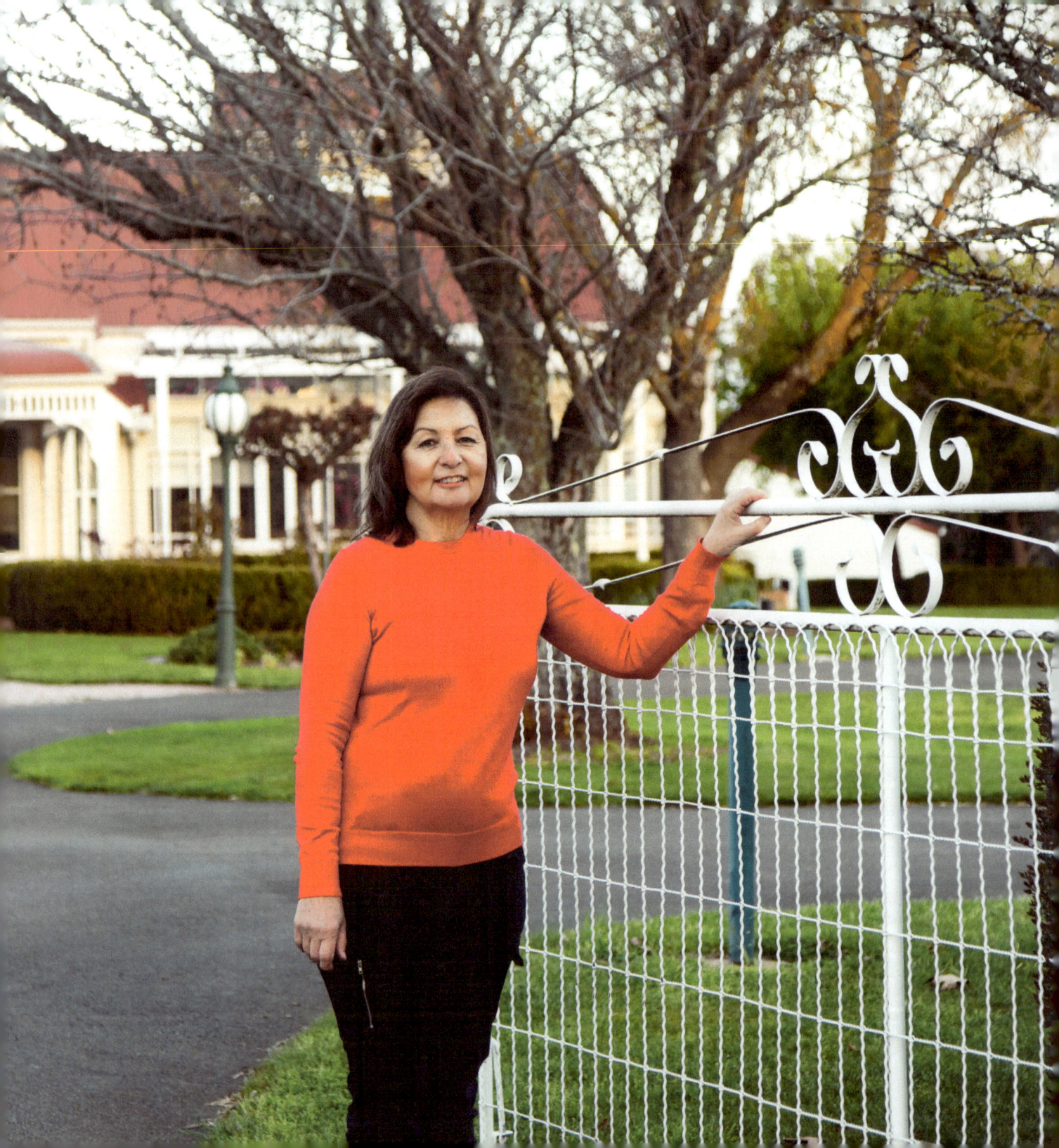

Introduction

The creation of *Nutritious and Delicious* has become the most wondrously unexpected adventure of all my forays into cooking. It all began from the most inspiring, professional experience I undertook in 2019 with Leiths School of Food and Wine in the United Kingdom, one of the most prestigious cooking schools in the UK. Travelling to London to complete the final exam of Leiths Essential Cooking Course was an exciting achievement in my long passion for healthy food and cooking. I became so captivated by the sagacity my culinary journey was unearthing that despite the world dealing with a pandemic, I was able to further my studies and undertake Leiths Nutrition in Culinary Practice Course remotely.

This experience was a watershed for me in learning how to incorporate in depth nutrition principles with well-balanced food options. I have integrated and expanded on these values in this book to provide lush and luxuriant meal options that anyone can master for a healthy meal or nourishing snack that fulfils our temptations and our bodies' needs any time of the day.

For many months I studied, cooked and photographed each tantalizing recipe from my own homestead kitchen in the fertile Strathbogie Ranges, modifying and experimenting to ultimately develop a versatile resource of recipes for people looking to prioritise both nutrition and taste. Our innate sense of nutrition and health is often thwarted by packaged convenience in today's attitude to food. This is the book that reasserts that knowledge from a new modern perspective.

This outlook has opened a window for me to share with others the ease, pleasure and benefit of putting nutrition at the forefront of every meal while emphasising seasonal flavours and discovering new taste combinations. This is possible for everyone: individuals and families in every setting as long as the right planning is undertaken first. These recipes use simple and wholesome ingredients that maximise the nutrition potential with delightful textures and flavours.

Previously my husband and I had enjoyed the rewards of running a small yet very successful vineyard in the Yarra Valley before fate encouraged us to move to a self-sustaining property in 2010 only a few hours from Melbourne. We were both products of a concrete jungle growing up in the suburbs of Melbourne so were always eager to live on the land, firstly by chance through viticulture and then turning our hands to extensive farming on our new property.

My working-class parents arrived from Poland in 1951 and scrimped and saved for our family for many years. My mother cooked from necessity rather than a love of it; nevertheless, standing beside her in our warm kitchen, talking and learning the dishes of her homeland, planted my lifelong love of cooking and all it represents; family, living well and being close to nature.

Over the years I dabbled in cooking classes and formal courses, loving the process of learning about new ingredients and menu ideas on a humble yet practical scale. My love of cooking (and particularly of healthy finger food) had proven an asset with our vineyard enterprise, as we expanded to host functions and weddings and the pairing of good food and wine became a fine art that I loved developing.

I have always sought out exotic new cuisines and was seduced by the light fresh flavours of Vietnam many years ago. Following the culinary trails of such a vibrant country saw my love for this well-balanced, healthy cuisine grow eternally. I completed fabulous regional cooking courses while I was there in order to discover the secrets of their distinctive fish sauce, and how their aromatic herbs and subtle spices create full flavoured dishes that satisfy so many of our dietary needs.

I now grow many of these unique Vietnamese herbs in my hothouse, and my extensive kitchen garden is a treasure trove of seasonal crops. I have a particular penchant for braised cabbage, an ode to my Polish heritage. My father's passion was tending the veggie garden in our backyard; it was his haven. He spent precious time with me in the garden when I was very young teaching me how to collect and dry seeds for the next planting. After school I would snack on fresh tomatoes, cucumbers and strawberries as I wandered through the garden waiting for my parents to arrive home from work.

Just like in my father's day, planting, growing and being self-sufficient is an important part of healthy living. Home vegetable gardens are sustainable, don't use

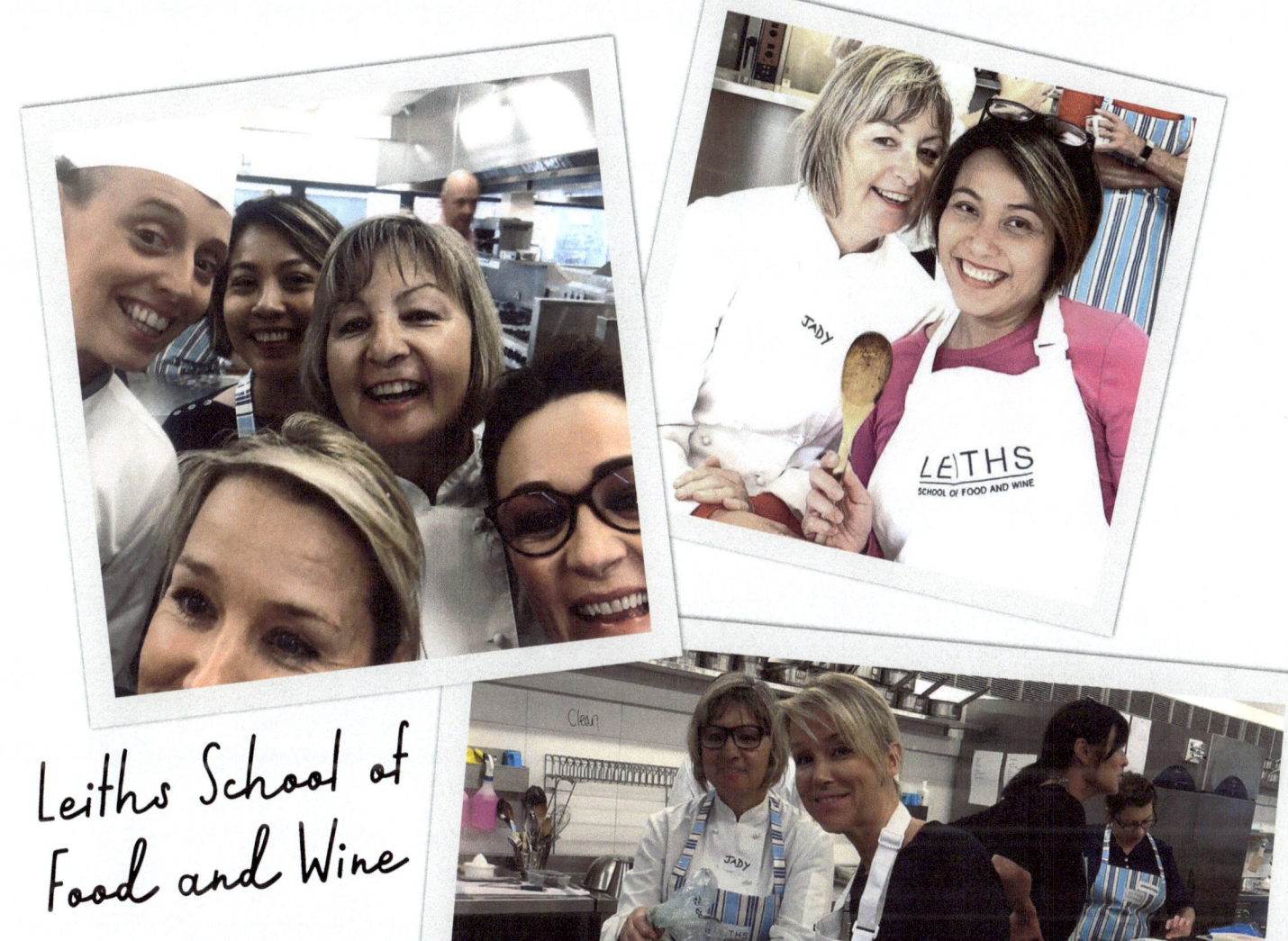

Leiths School of Food and Wine

pesticides and provide the freshest produce straight into your kitchen. When there is a bumper harvest the surplus can be frozen for use in non-seasonal times, preserved or shared with family, friends, or the local community. Fresh home-grown produce is without doubt the best because the nutritional value of fruit and vegetables starts to wane upon harvest so growing your own or buying from a local farmers' market benefits you and so many others in the community.

Self-seeding plants are great too in saving you time and money. Having a vegetable garden is not only sustainable but also fun; digging, planting and caring for your garden gives endless pleasure as well as the benefit of exercising out in the fresh air. I love each moment of the many hours I tend my garden just as my father did.

I have loved passing on this legacy to our grandchildren who know where their food is grown. They know food isn't meant to have pesticides or wasteful packaging. Their visits are full of joy as they run to the chook house to collect the eggs, dash off to munch in the raspberry and strawberry patch before they carefully collect the ripe produce from the kitchen garden and show it to me proudly.

My love of cooking using home grown ingredients has ignited my humble expectations of simply studying and cooking during the pandemic into a tinderbox of inspiration. Unlocking the potential of *Nutritious and Delicious* for people that have a similar impetus to learn more about easy, healthy cooking but don't quite know where to begin. I am now stirred to action, and I am in the process of opening up our cottage doors to cooking classes and farm stays, to welcome like-minded people who are at the start of their cookery and nutrition adventure.

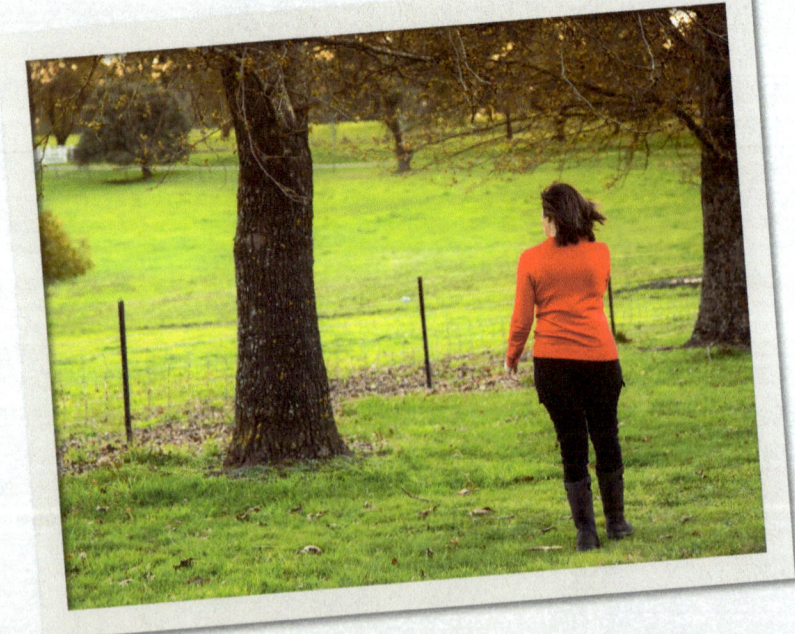

You don't need to feel like a natural cook, we can get you there with your enthusiasm for health and nutrition and by following along as you build up your knowledge and understanding of fulfilling our bodies' dietary needs. It is heartening to know we can improve our wellbeing and that of our loved-ones, by embracing wholesome foods and recipes that are as beautiful as they are *Nutritious and Delicious*, enjoy!

The Fundamentals of *Nutritious and Delicious*

The fundamentals behind the recipes in this book are based on ingredients in their most natural form, and then combining these nutrients to create simple yet delicious flavours that will change the way you approach food forever.

Healthy eating begins with organisational planning and preparation. Rethinking how you shop, stock your pantry and prepare food can provide your family and friends with *Nutritious and Delicious* meals.

Before you get busy in the kitchen though, let's highlight some very important nutrition principles to a healthy diet. Once you get the hang of how easy it is to combine nutrition with immense flavour, you'll incorporate these principles effortlessly into your lifestyle.

Nutrition

Good nutrition is about consuming natural foods that contain important nutrients for our energy output and our body's internal functions. There are seven main classes of nutrients that the body needs on a daily basis to help us build and maintain health and wellbeing:

- Carbohydrates
- Protein
- Fats
- Vitamins
- Minerals
- Fibre
- Water

Carbohydrates, Protein and Fats (along with Water) are referred to as macronutrients and are the main pillars of a healthy diet. Macronutrients make up most of our daily nutritional needs, more than 80% in fact.

MACRONUTRIENT	RECOMMENDED DIETARY INTAKE IN AUSTRALIA[1]
Carbohydrates	45-65 % of daily intake
Protein	15-25 % of daily intake
Fats	20-35 % of daily intake
Water	2-3 litres per day for adults

---

[1] Grech, Amanda et al. 'Macronutrient Composition of the Australian Population's Diet; Trends from Three National Nutrition Surveys 1983, 1995 and 2012.' *Nutrients* vol. 10,8 1045. 8 Aug. 2018, doi:10.3390/nu10081048

Micronutrients are the vitamins and minerals found in whole food sources and while they're vital for strong bones and healthy blood cells etc., they are needed in smaller amounts. In today's busy lifestyle supplements are available however nature provides them in the perfect quality and amount and so these are not needed in a well balanced diet.

NUTRITION TIPS

Keep in mind these little tips as you shop, snack and prepare meals.

- Aim for seasonally available fresh fruit and vegetables for optimal quality and nutrition.
- Fresh raw food maintains the most nutrients.
- For texture, flavour and mouthfeel use a variety of vegetables and herbs on your plate.
- A rainbow of colours on your plate ensures a range of vitamins and minerals.
- Use herbs, nuts and seeds as an ingredient rather than a garnish.
- Use fresh herbs and spices to flavour and season food in lieu of too much salt and sugar.
- Cook with healthy fats, which you will learn about as you read on.

Let's explore macro and micro nutrients a little further because understanding the nutritional constructs of food will help you to confidently reach for healthy choices for your meals and snacks each day, as well as for your loved-ones.

Carbohydrates

WHAT YOU NEED TO KNOW

Carbohydrates are a major macronutrient and your body's main source of energy providing important vitamins, minerals and fibre. They help fuel your brain, kidneys, heart muscles, and central nervous system.

Carbohydrates are found in many different plant foods, and it's generally recommended they make up between 45-65% of your diet. It's important to know that carbohydrates come in two forms (complex and simple) and maintaining a healthy diet is about eating the *right* carbohydrates.

Complex carbohydrates are natural, unprocessed foods known for releasing energy into the body slowly (as they contain more fibre), which helps to keep you full for longer.

Sources of complex carbohydrates include:

- Fruit
- Vegetables
- Whole grains/seeds
- Brown and wild rice
- Nuts
- Legumes

Simple (or refined) carbohydrates contain far less fibre so they are released into the bloodstream quickly after eating, leading to a spike in blood sugar. Simple carbohydrates should be reduced in your daily intake.

Sources of simple carbohydrates include:

- White bread
- White rice
- White pasta
- Soft drinks
- Concentrated juices
- Breakfast cereals
- Baked items

For a healthy diet more complex carbohydrates should be consumed than simple carbohydrates, this provides optimal macronutrients and better blood sugar management.

Protein

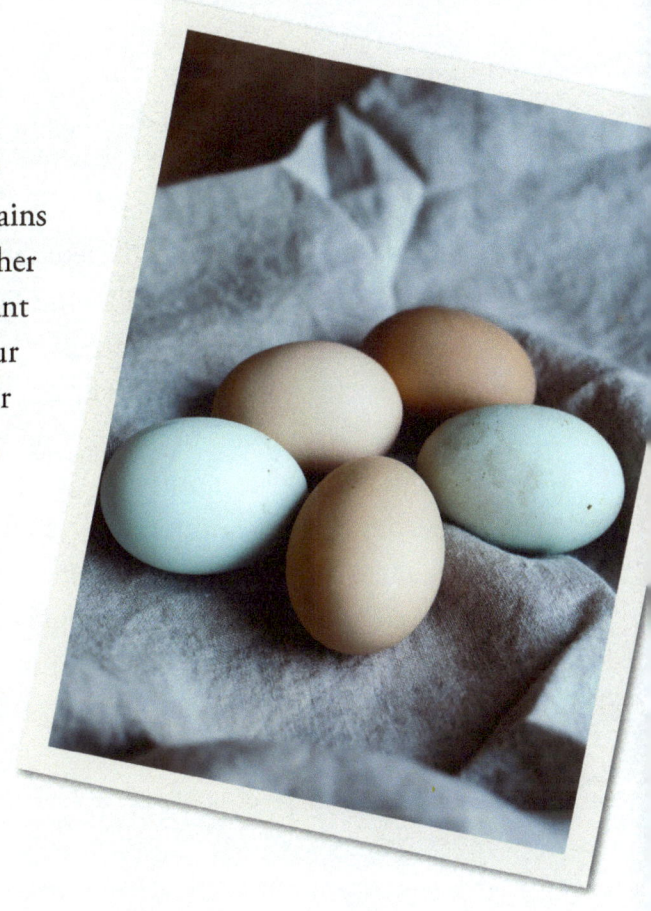

GREAT FOR HEALTH AND FITNESS

Every cell in the human body contains protein, that's why it is considered another macronutrient that we need significant amounts of each day. Protein helps our body to build, replenish, and repair tissues and organs. Our bones, nails, hair, muscles and genetic materials all need protein.

More specifically, protein is a compound made up of 22 amino acids that the body needs. 9 of these are considered essential because our body cannot produce them. So it's good to eat protein from a variety of plant and animal sources to get a good balance of amino acids.

Our body cannot store protein the way carbohydrates and fats are stored, so if we don't eat enough protein our body starts to break down muscle mass. The recommended daily intake of protein is between 10-35% of our total calories.

Foods rich in protein include:

- Eggs
- Chicken
- Dairy products
- Oats
- Almonds
- Meat
- Lentils
- Soybeans

One of the few plant-based foods that contain all 9 essential amino acids is quinoa. It's gluten free and contains more iron, zinc, fibre and magnesium than most grains. Quinoa can be boiled and makes a delicious porridge.

Chia seeds contain a lot of protein as well as omega-3 fatty acids (essential), calcium, magnesium, selenium and iron. Chia seeds absorb liquid and form a gel, which means they are great for thickening jams and stewed fruit.

Beans are one of the healthiest foods to eat. In addition to protein, beans contain good amounts of fibre keeping you fuller for longer, and your cholesterol levels low. Beans are great for breakfast, in soups or salads, and when pureed can be used to thicken sauce. Using beans to create a dip makes for a healthy choice.

Peanut butter is also another plant-based protein. You can put a tablespoon on some apple or pear for a healthy snack or add it to smoothies, curries and sauces to name a few. To maintain a feeling of fullness for longer, try and eat protein at every meal or snack time.

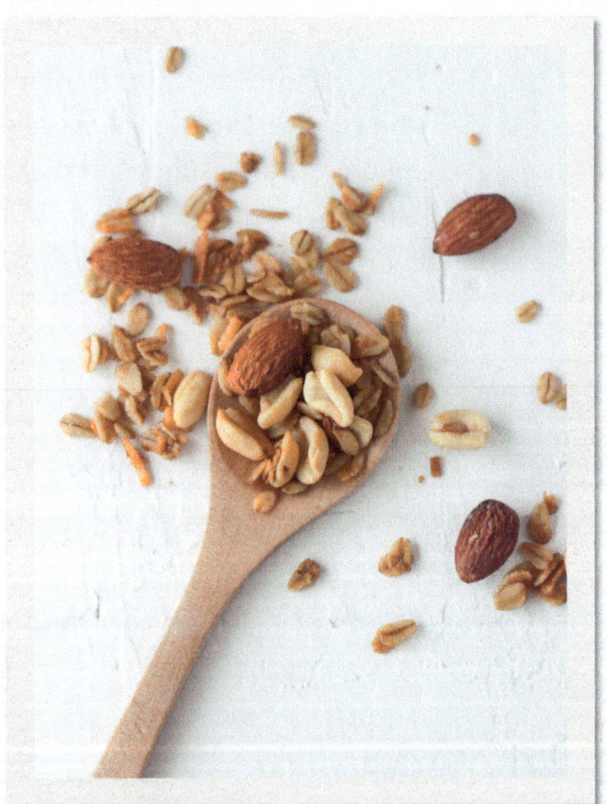

Fats

The third main building block (or macronutrient) in nutrition is fat, or more specifically, good fats. Fats provide us with energy, add flavor and importantly support cell growth, provide internal warmth and also protect our organs. Fats should be included in moderation in a healthy diet as they are high in calories.

Fats come from animal (e.g. beef, pork, poultry, lamb, butter, milk, cream) and plant sources (olives, avocados, vegetable oils, coconut, soybean, nuts and seeds). Vitamins from fats can be either water-soluble which move through the body quickly, or fat-soluble such as Vitamins A, D, E and K. These vitamins require fat for absorption and are stored in fatty tissues in the body.

There are four types of fats to be aware of:

1. Unsaturated fats (monounsaturated and polyunsaturated)
2. Saturated fats
3. Cholesterol
4. Trans fats

Unsaturated fats are liquid at room temperature. Good sources of monounsaturated fats are found in olive oil, grapeseed oil, peanut oil and avocado oil. Sources of polyunsaturated fats include safflower seeds, flax seeds, tahini, nuts and safflower oil.

Unsaturated fats are also a good source of essential fats and oils that our body needs but cannot produce itself; these are known as omega-3 and omega-6 fats. They have a range of health benefits including heart health, insulating nerve fibres, lowering blood pressure, supporting our immune system and reducing inflammation.

Sources of omega-3:

- Oily fish (salmon, sardines etc.)
- Soybeans
- Nuts
- Eggs
- Dairy
- Seeds (flax, chia etc.)
- Green vegetables (spinach, kale etc.)

Sources of omega-6:

- Vegetable oils
- Meat
- Eggs
- Avocados
- Nuts
- Whole grains
- Peanut butter
- Tofu

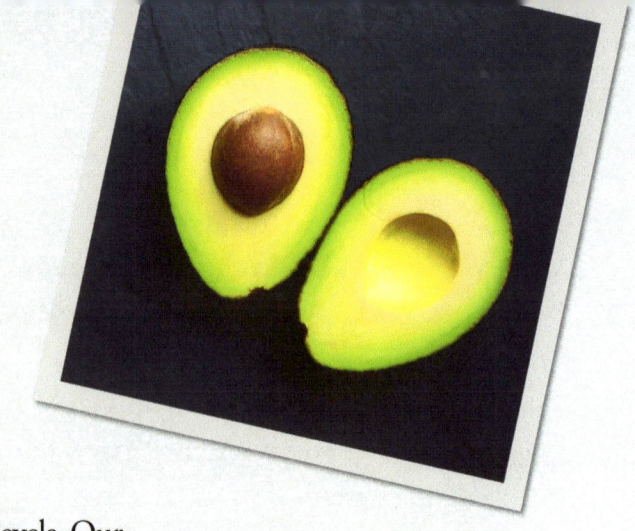

CHOLESTEROL

It's important to understand how consuming saturated fats and trans fats can affect your cholesterol levels. Our body produces enough of its own cholesterol for important bodily functions, so it is a non-essential nutrient (we do not have to look for it in food sources). Consuming food with cholesterol can increase our cholesterol to unhealthy levels.

There are two forms of cholesterol to identify in food: low density lipoprotein (LDL) and high density lipoprotein (HDL), and they act very differently in our body! LDL has a high proportion of cholesterol to protein which means cholesterol is deposited into the arteries sometimes damaging and/or blocking them. Think of LDL as bad cholesterol.

HDL has a higher proportion of protein to cholesterol, they actually move through the blood stream picking up excess cholesterol and depositing them into the liver for disposal. Think of HDL as good cholesterol.

SATURATED AND TRANS FATS

Saturated fats are solid at room temperature. Red meat and dairy are two common sources of saturated fats although nuts and seeds contain a small percentage of saturated fats as well.

Most of the trans fats we consume are created through a process called hydrogenation that makes the existing liquid fats and oils *more saturated* or solid. This is helpful for food manufacturers as cheaper oils can be used and greater saturation extends the shelf life of products.

Hydrogenation occurs in processed foods and produces more LDLs, that's the important bit to remember so you can learn to avoid them!

LDL foods to avoid:

- Fatty cuts of meats
- Bacon, sausages etc.
- Cured meats
- Deep fried food
- Fast food
- Biscuits/cakes
- Pastries/pies

HDL foods to eat:

- Olive oil
- Eggs
- Avocado
- Beans
- Legumes
- Whole grains
- Oily fish
- Nuts
- Chia seeds

The recommended daily intake of fats should be 20-30% of total calories.[2] Omega-3 and omega-6 sources are the most beneficial.

COOKING WITH OILS

The smoke point of cooking oils is important to know because the smoke gives off toxic fumes and creates harmful free radicals to humans.

Smoke points vary greatly but in general, the more refined an oil, the higher its smoke point. Refined oils typically have a neutral taste and odour and a clearer appearance. Light olive oil for example has been refined and has a higher smoke point (240°C) whereas extra virgin olive oil (190°C) has not been refined and is not neutral in taste.

High smoke point oils begin at 205°C, some of these include, light olive oil, vegetable, rice bran, peanut, sunflower and safflower oils. These oils are neutral and won't taint the taste of food.

Unrefined oils such as walnut, argan and hemp seed oil have a low smoke point

---

[2] Liu, Ann G et al. 'A healthy approach to dietary fats: understanding the science and taking action to reduce consumer confusion.' *Nutrition journal* vol. 16,1 53. 30 Aug. 2017, doi:10.1186/s12937-017-0271-4

and should not be heated. Use for cooler recipes such as dressings, sauces, smoothies and dips.

Coconut oil is a type of saturated fat however it is absorbed directly into the liver for energy rather than fat storage so it is generally considered safe to use in cooking in moderate amounts.

Store oils in a cool, dark cupboard or the refrigerator. This prevents the oil from going rancid. Buying oil in small quantities is good practice as oils go rancid after six months of opening. Some oils stored in the refrigerator turn cloudy. Once brought back to room temperature oils will return to original consistency and are safe to consume.

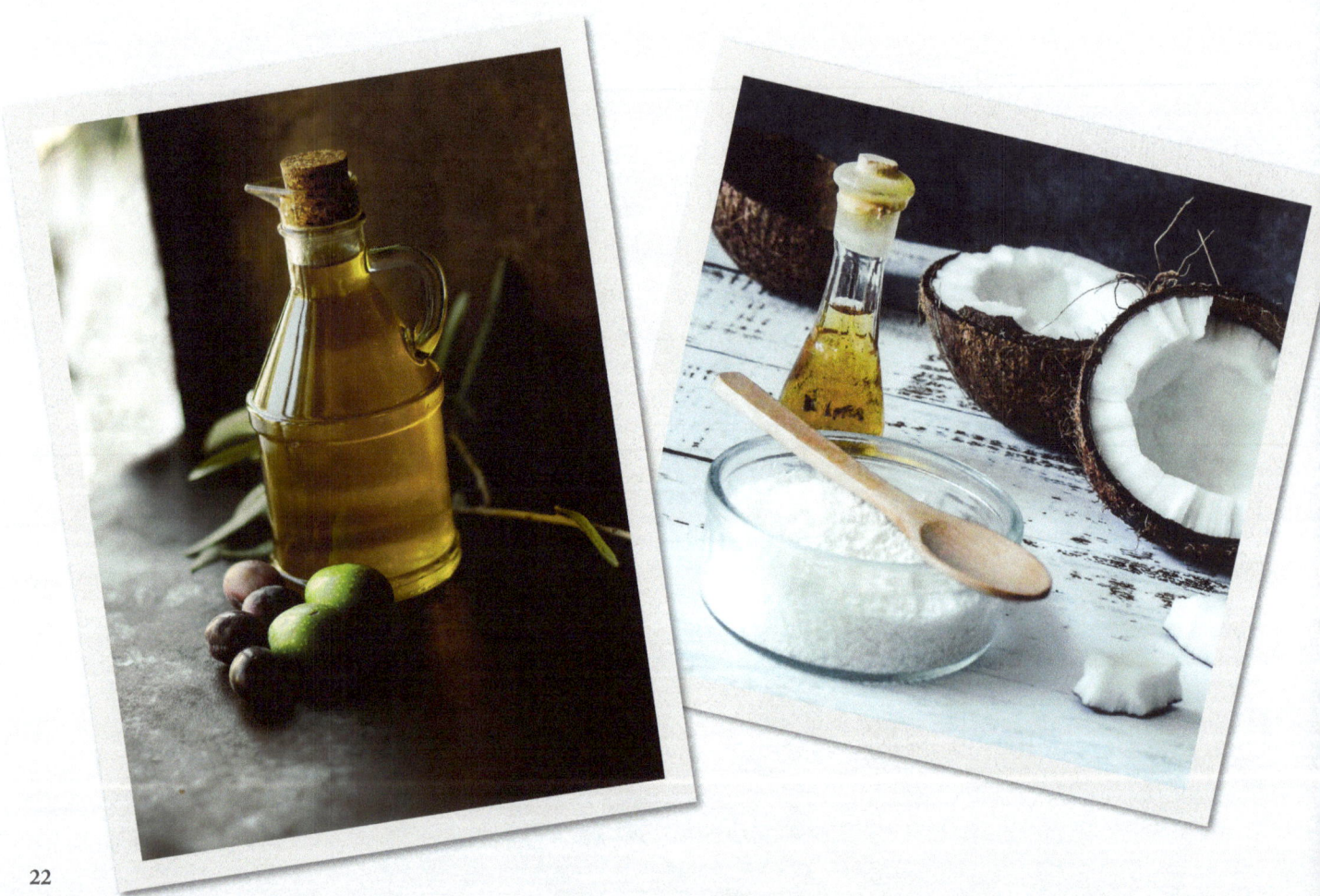

Fibre

WHAT'S THE DEAL?

Fibre is the buzz word of recent decades – we're always being asked, "Are you getting enough fibre in your diet?" But not everyone knows what it actually is or what it does for us.

Fibre is a type of carbohydrate found in plants – it gives them their firm structure. Fibre is made up of indigestible compounds, which pass relatively unchanged through our body, keeping our digestive system healthy.

There are three types of fibre: soluble, insoluble and resistant starch:

Soluble fibre absorbs water and forms a gel in our gut. This helps us to feel full and it feeds our gut bacteria. Foods that are high in soluble fibre are legumes, oats, barley and citrus fruit.

Insoluble fibre provides us with dietary roughage which also makes us feel full and promotes bowel movement. Foods that are high in insoluble fibre are brown rice, root vegetables, skins, seeds and seeds of fruit, nuts and legumes.

Resistant starch is formed when starch-containing foods are cooked and cooled, such as rice. It occurs due to retrogradation, which refers to the collective processes of dissolved starch becoming less soluble after being heated, dissolved in water and then cooled. That food then becomes more resistant to digestion. Foods that contain resistant starch are beans, peas, lentils, oats, barley, cooked and cooled rice, potatoes and pasta.

Resistant starch acts as a prebiotic which feeds our good gut bacteria. So how do we get resistant starch into our diet? Cook rice, pasta or potatoes the day before. Cool, refrigerate and consume the next day. Reheating the food will still retain the same qualities.

Soaking oats, quinoa, chia seeds with milk or yoghurt overnight and eating the following day is a great way to get resistant starch into your diet. Freezing bananas, for example, turns starch into resistant starch.

Vitamins & Minerals

Vitamins and minerals are micronutrients that perform so many important roles in the body to help us develop and stay healthy. Vitamins assist with wound healing, boosting immunity, repairing cellular damage and converting food into energy.

Minerals are needed for the formation and composition of bones, blood and teeth, and the maintenance of normal cell and nerve function.

Vitamins and minerals are required in small amounts but interestingly our body cannot produce them so we must obtain them in our food sources. The exception to this rule is Vitamin D, which our body can produce when exposed to direct sunlight.

Vitamins can be either fat-soluble or water-soluble. Fat-soluble vitamins (vitamins A, D, E and K) dissolve in fats and oils (not water), and can be stored in fatty tissue. While water soluble vitamins are utilised as they pass through the body.

Fat-soluble vitamins:

- Vitamin A (retinol) is important for vision, immunity, skin, nerve cells and thyroid activity. It is found in eggs, dairy, oily fish, liver as well as in orange-coloured fruits and vegetables.

- Vitamin D regulates calcium and phosphate for healthy bones and teeth. It is produced by sunlight and found in small amounts in foods such as oily fish, egg yolks, liver and red meat.

- Vitamin E is an antioxidant and helps maintain healthy skin and eyes. It is mainly found in plant oils, soya, sunflower seeds and wheat germ.

- Vitamin K plays a role in blood clotting and supporting our bones. It is mainly found in dark green leafy vegetables but also in small quantities in meat and dairy.

Water-soluble vitamins:

- Vitamin B plays a vital role in maintaining good health and wellbeing. Vitamin B has a direct impact on your energy levels, cell metabolism and brain function. Vitamin B is found in dairy, eggs, red meat, chicken, fish, shellfish, dark green vegetables, bananas and mushrooms.

- Vitamin C (ascorbic acid) is an essential nutrient for our immunity and is involved in repairing tissues. Vitamin C is found in citrus fruit, tomatoes, broccoli, kale, red capsicums and berries.

A rainbow of colours on your plate is not only visually appealing it has great health benefits too. Here are some of nature's coloured-coded health benefits:

- Blue/purple foods are extremely high in antioxidants e.g. blueberries, blackberries, grapes, beetroot, red cabbage and eggplant.
- Green foods are abundant in heart health nutrients e.g. kale, broccoli, cabbage and spinach.
- Orange foods are high in carotenoids. These compounds help provide Vitamin A, or retinol, to the body. Vitamin A helps us see at night, keeps our immune system strong and keeps our skin cells healthy e.g. carrots, oranges, pumpkin and sweet potato.
- Yellow foods contain large amounts of bioflavonoids, which help to reduce inflammation and fight infection e.g. lemon, ginger, turmeric and yellow capsicums.
- Red foods contain high levels of lycopene and anthocyanins, which are thought to be effective in bacterial infections, macular degeneration and neurological disease e.g. tomatoes, red capsicums, raspberries, pomegranate, rhubarb, strawberries and cherries.

Foods and their minerals to look for:

- Calcium is required for bones, teeth, and muscle contraction e.g. dark green leafy vegetables, almonds, tofu and sunflower seeds.

- Sodium helps with muscle and nerve function e.g. salt, avocado, celery, spinach, meat and dairy.
- Iron helps with the production of red blood cells e.g. beef, kale, broccoli and oats.
- Iodine helps with thyroid function e.g. shellfish, sea fish, milk, cheese and yoghurt.
- Fluoride prevents teeth decay e.g. black tea, coffee, mineral water, grapes, raisins and potatoes.
- Chromium regulates blood sugar and the breakdown of fats and carbohydrates e.g. rye bread, potatoes and apples.
- Phosphorus is required to build and repair bones and teeth, helps nerve function and muscle contraction e.g. dairy, meat, wholegrains, nuts, seeds and legumes.
- Magnesium helps with muscle and nerve function e.g. avocado, nuts, dark chocolate, legumes and seeds.
- Copper helps produce red and white blood cells e.g. nuts, seeds, organ meat, shiitake mushrooms and dark chocolate.
- Potassium plays a vital role in healthy heart, kidney, muscle and nerve function. Potassium and sodium regulate fluid balance and are necessary for a healthy heart, e.g. avocado, kiwi fruit, bananas, potato, and sundried tomatoes.
- Zinc supports proper immune system function, skin health, prostate and fertility, e.g. eggs, dairy, legumes, nuts, seeds, ginger and oysters.

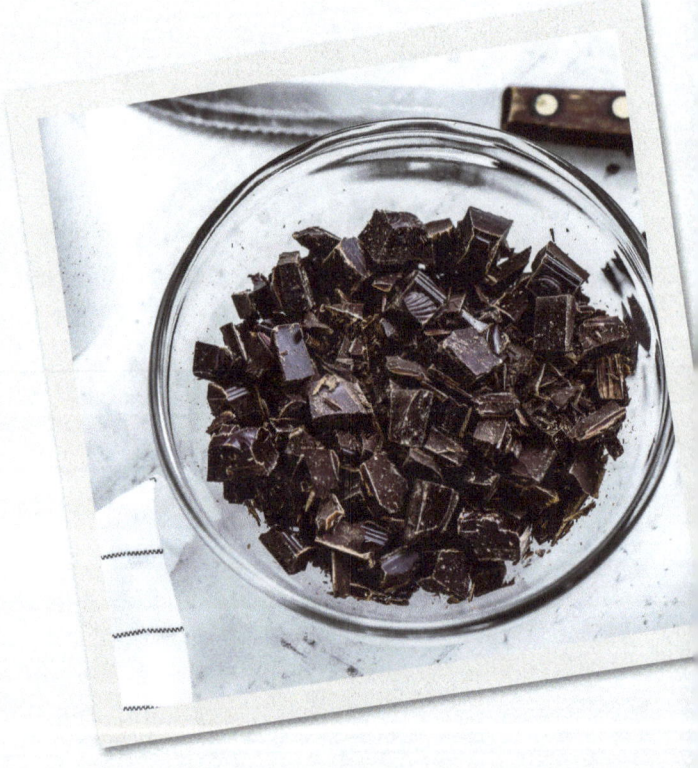

Grains

Since hunter-gatherer times, grains have been an integral part of the human diet and an important source of macronutrients. Whole grains are good sources of fibre. Fibre takes longer to digest resulting in a slow steady release of glucose in the bloodstream. Eating refined grains such as white rice and pasta result in quick surges of blood glucose soon after eating so feelings of hunger return sooner.

Healthy whole grains include:

- Oats are high in fibre, keeping you full longer and a great food to include in your breakfast routine. Overnight oats can be made easily and stored for five days in the refrigerator.

- Bulgur wheat is a fibre-rich whole grain that is nutrient dense. It contains protein and B vitamins.

- Barley is a cereal grain with a chewy texture and nutty flavour. It's rich in vitamins and minerals and has a high fibre content which lessens feelings of hunger.

- Quinoa is high in protein. It has all 9 essential amino acids making it a complete protein. Quinoa consists of insoluble fibre and resistant starch. Quinoa is gluten free and has a low Glycemic Index.

- Brown rice has the hull removed leaving the nutrient packed bran and germ. Brown rice retains vitamins, minerals and antioxidants. It's a good source of vitamin B2, potassium, calcium and manganese.

Herbs and Spices

Herbs and spices are a great source of nutrition. They're cultivated for their aromatic properties, pungency and nutritional and medicinal qualities. They are also low in calories and are a great way to introduce additional nutrients into your daily intake. Spices and herbs have been used since ancient times to add flavour to food and contribute colours and variety. Spices and herbs can also reduce the need for salt and sugar in food.

Herbs are usually the leaves of the plant, and include rosemary, basil, sage, thyme, oregano, parsley and coriander. Herbs are packed with important nutrients and antioxidants. Incorporating herbs can transform every meal, making it nutritious and delicious. Just like leafy green vegetables, fresh herbs contain large amounts of vitamins A, C and K.

- Herbs such as coriander are good sources of vitamins A, C, K and E, and may help fight infections and reduce inflammation.

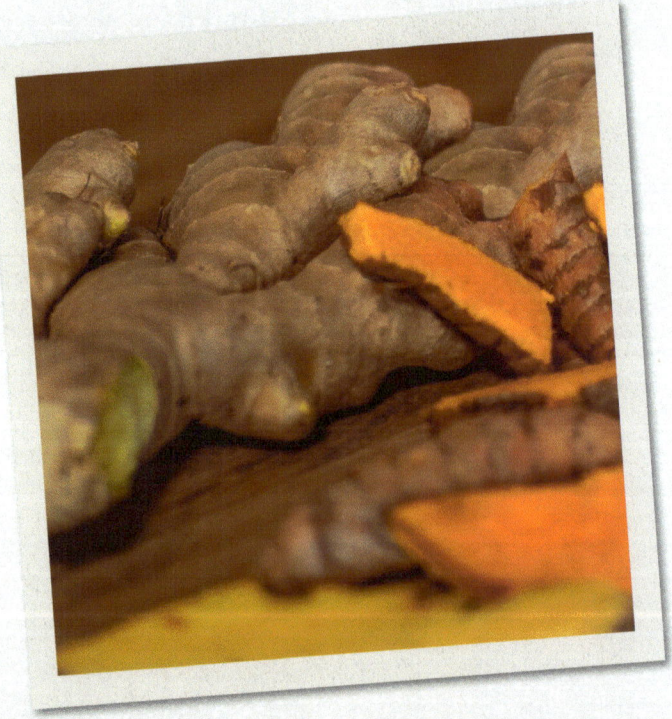

Spices come from the non-leafy parts of the plant, including roots, bark, berries, flowers and seeds. For example, cinnamon is a bark, ginger and turmeric are roots, peppercorns are berries, cardamon is a pod or seed and cloves are flower buds. Spices have many health benefits:

- Turmeric and ginger are good for the immune system.
- Cinnamon can help lower blood sugar.
- Peppercorns have anti-inflammatory properties.

Glycaemic Index

Glycaemic Index (GI) measures how carbohydrates affect blood sugar levels. This is measured on a scale of 1 to 100, heading up to the highest sugar level.

Foods with high and low GI affect blood sugar (glucose) differently. High GI foods make blood sugar rise and fall more quickly. On the other hand, low GI foods are absorbed more slowly when digested, so they take longer to enter the bloodstream and raise blood sugar at a much slower rate. This slow release of blood sugar into the bloodstream is much more beneficial, because it maintains our energy levels better and has many other health benefits. Lower GI foods often contain protein and/or fat, and are usually higher in fibre.

Valid scientific methods are used to measure the GI values of foods:

Low GI	55 or less
Mid GI	56 to 69
High GI	70+

Eating foods containing carbohydrates, the organic compounds that our bodies break down into glucose, affects how your blood sugar rises and falls. How high blood sugar rises and how long it stays high for depends on the GI as well as the quantity, measured in Glycaemic Load (GL). GL combines the quantity and the value (GI).

Low GL	10 or less
Mid GL	11 to 19
High GL	20 or more

To figure out the GL of a food, we can use the GL formula:

GL = (GI x carbohydrate grams per portion)/100

For example, one banana has a GI of 52 and has 16g of carbohydrates. So, 52 x 16/100 = 8.32. This means a banana has a low GL.

If you're consuming 2000 calories per day, it's recommended that you should target 100g of GL.

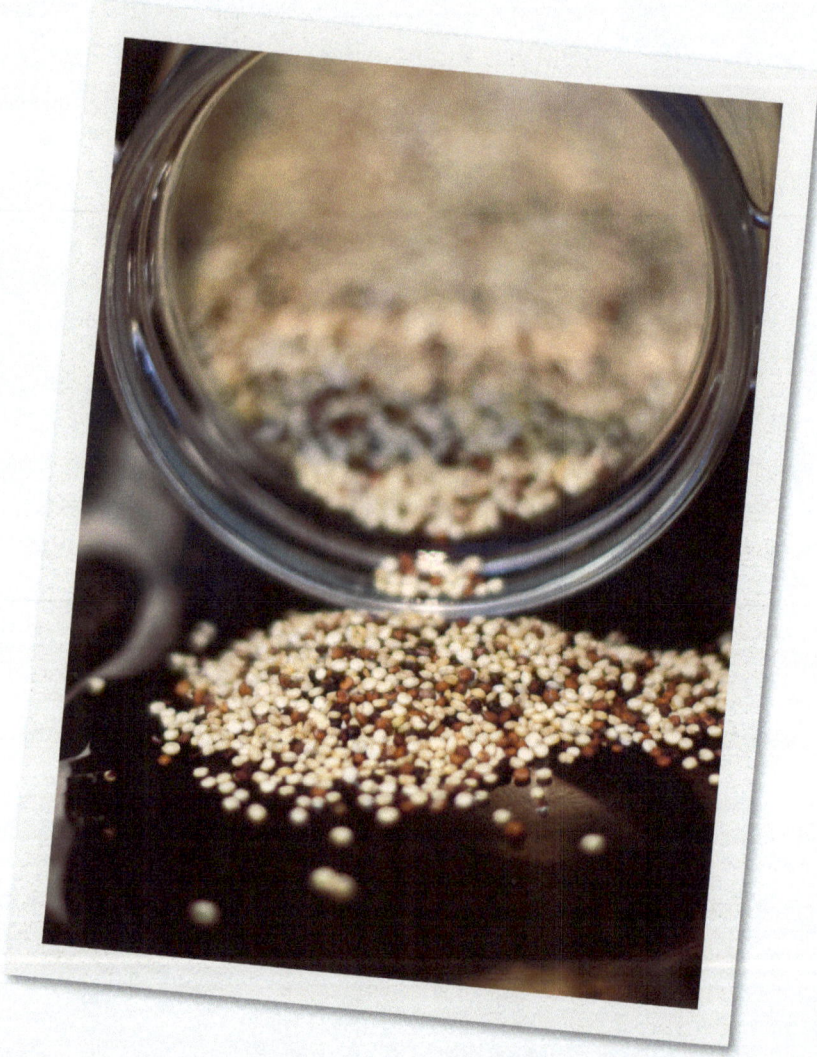

Planning Ahead

Learning to be organised is the key to preparing healthy meals. Being organised allows you to prepare healthy meals in less time. You can plan your meals and write them down to create visual reminders. While you're preparing to make a meal, thoroughly read the recipe to familiarise yourself with the techniques, equipment and ingredients you'll need. Prepare a shopping list based on ingredients you'll need, and shop accordingly. Only buy what you need, because healthy food begins with freshness.

Think ahead so you can prepare healthy meals in less time:

- Make breakfast in advance – overnight oats or chia can be made up to five days in advance.
- Cook your grains and let cool; then you can store in individual containers in the fridge for 3-5 days.
- Dressings can be made up to a week in advance.
- Proteins can be cooked in advance and prepared as a meal with grains, vegetables and dressing.
- Chop vegetables and store them in the fridge, ready for cooking or eating.

Portion Control

Even when eating healthy foods, we can eat more than our body requires. To determine how much you should be eating for optimal health and avoid overeating, use the size and width of your palm as a guide for portion control.

Keeping in mind the key macronutrients that should be consumed in most meals, when plating your meal, use the following 'rule of palm' formula:

- One palm-size portion each of protein and carbohydrates
- Two palm-size portions of fruit/vegetables
- Fat: half a thumb size

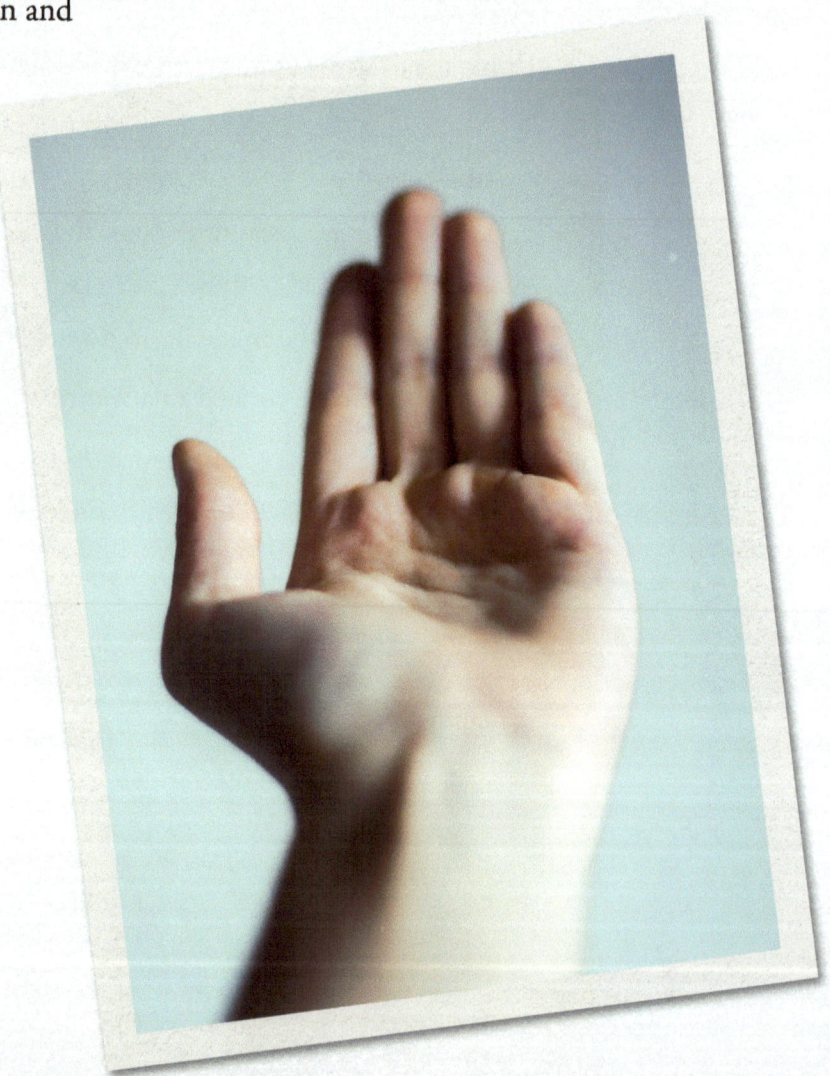

Pre and Probiotics

The World Health Organization defines pre- and probiotics as "Live micro-organisms which when administered in adequate amounts confer a benefit to the host."[3]

Probiotics contain bacteria and other micro-organisms, such as yeasts, in the gut microflora. These provide health benefits to the host, so they are often called 'good' bacteria. Foods containing probiotics include yoghurt, kefir, kimchi, kombucha, sauerkraut, tempeh and miso.

Prebiotics are non-digestible foods that feed the good bacteria in our gut. Eating enough prebiotics helps our gut maintain enough healthy bacteria. Foods that feed our gut include vegetables and fruits such as garlic, leeks, bananas, asparagus, artichokes, onion and tomato, and whole grains, roots, and fermented dairy such as yoghurt, buttermilk, kefir and breast milk.

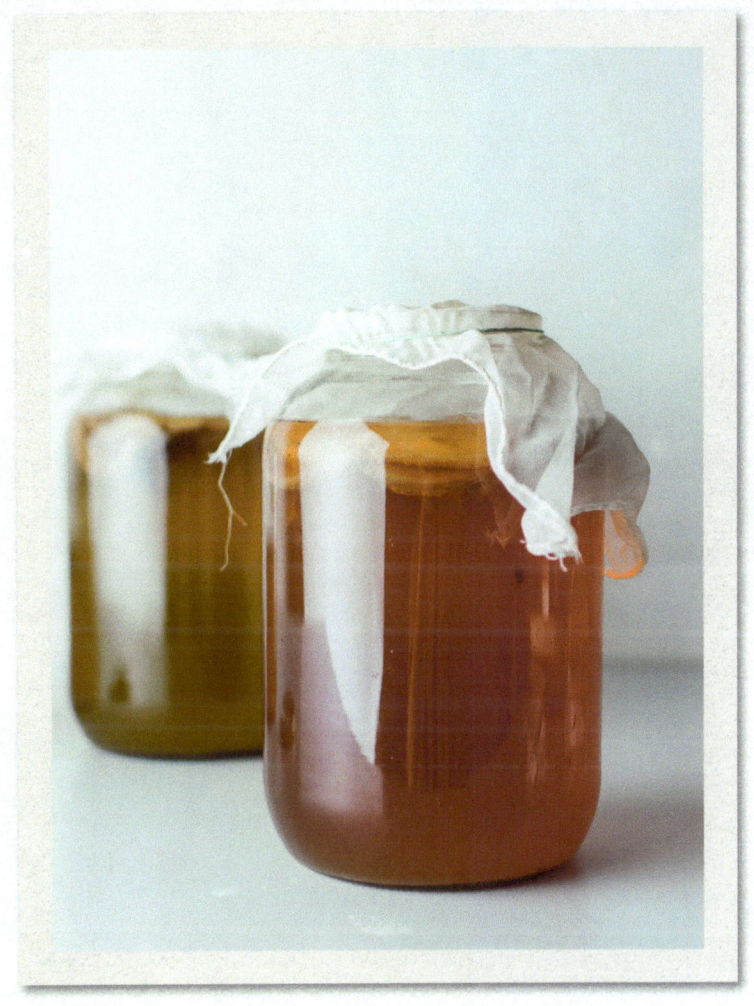

---

[3] World Health Organization and Food and Agriculture Organization of the United Nations, (2002) 'Guidelines for the Evaluation of Probiotics in Food', https://www.who.int/foodsafety/fs_management/en/probiotic_guidelines.pdf

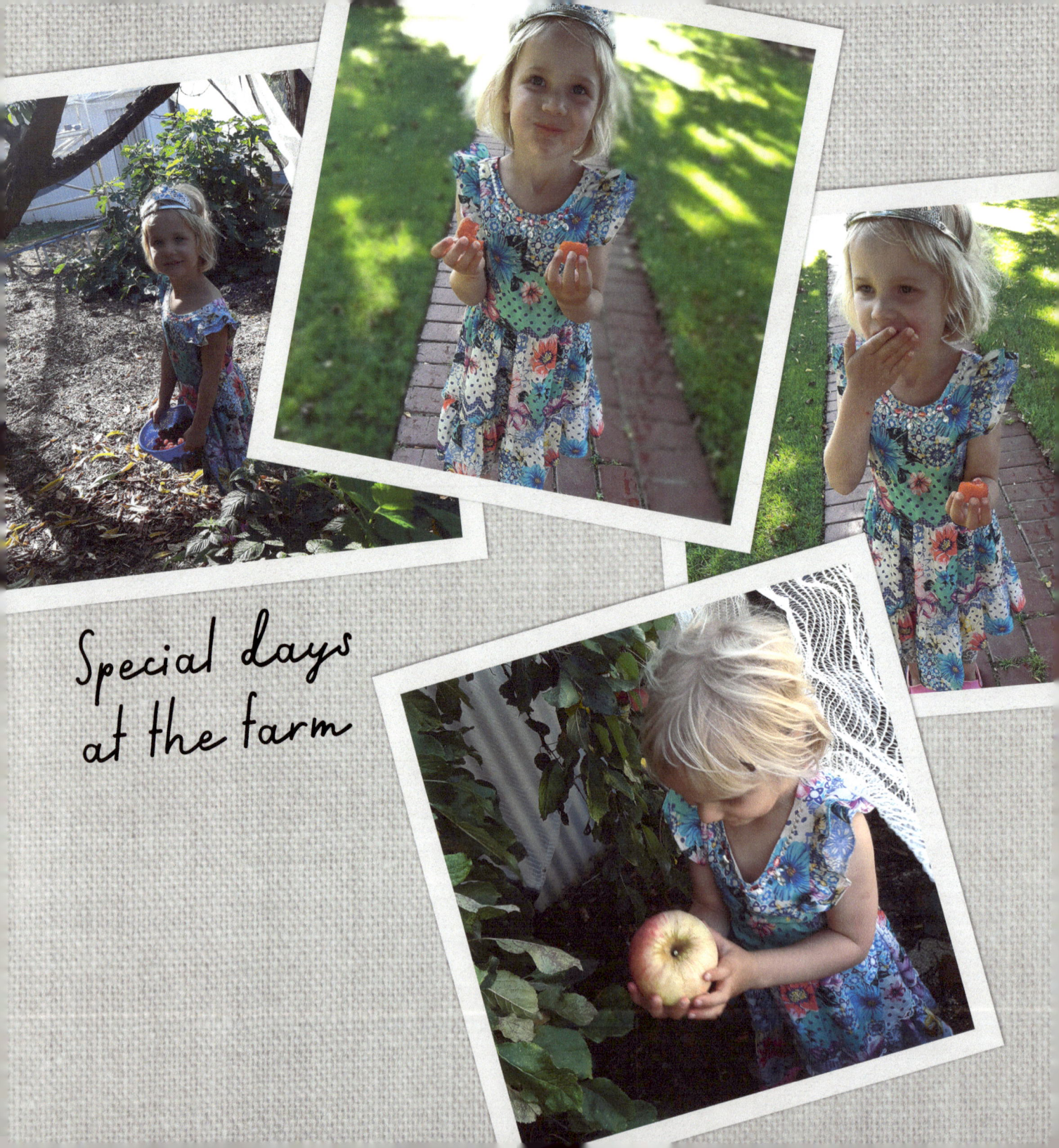
Special days at the farm

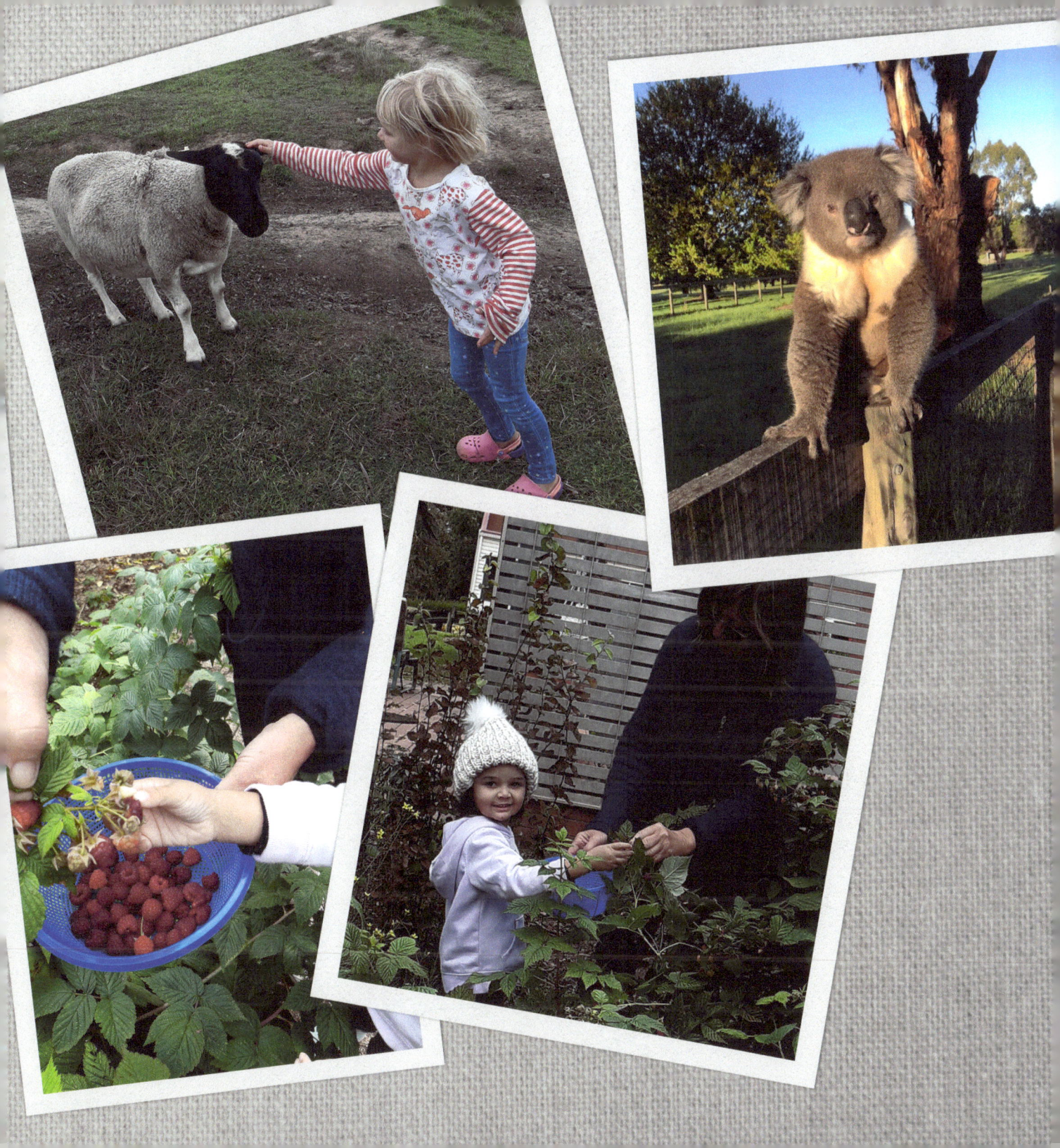

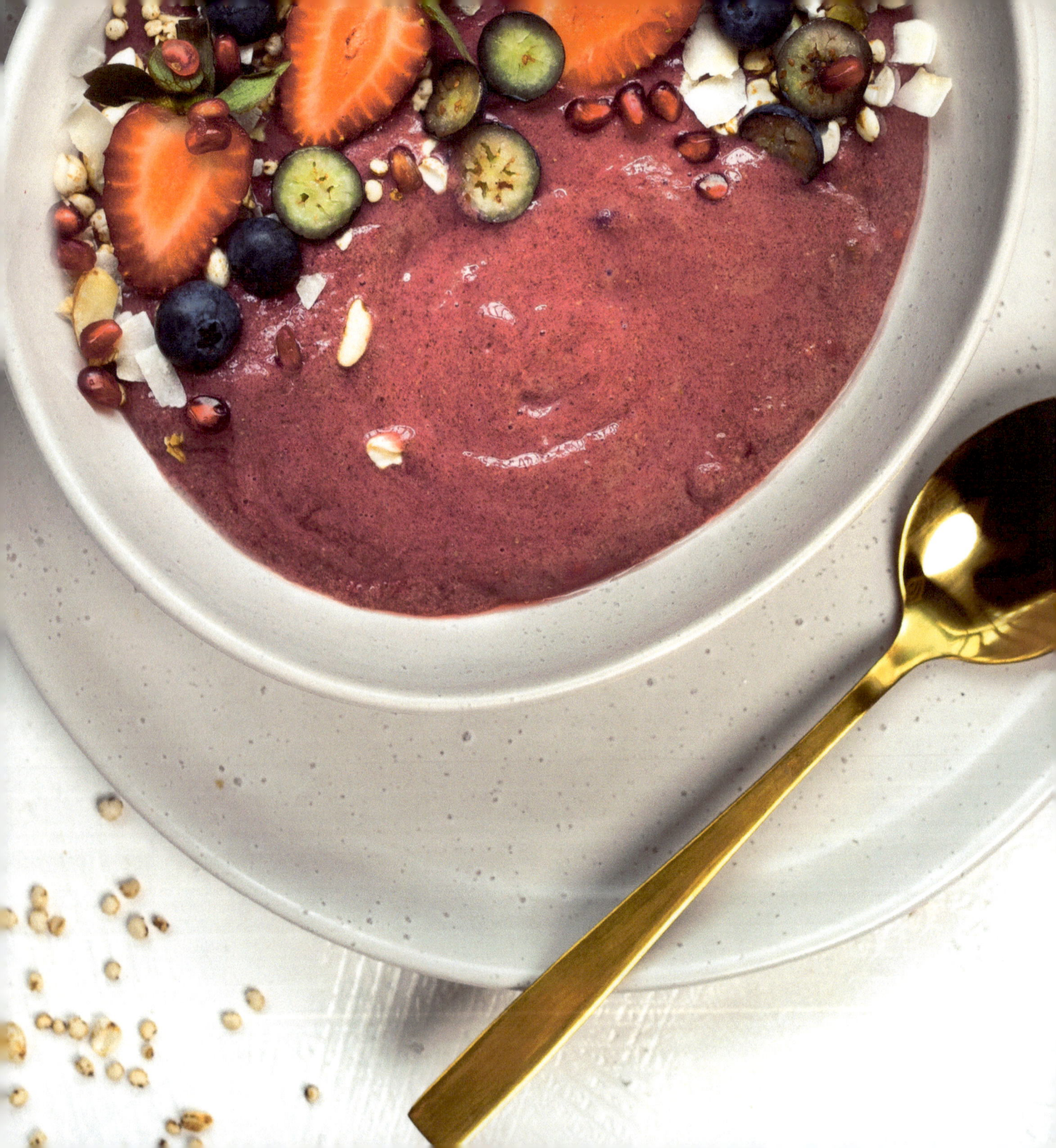

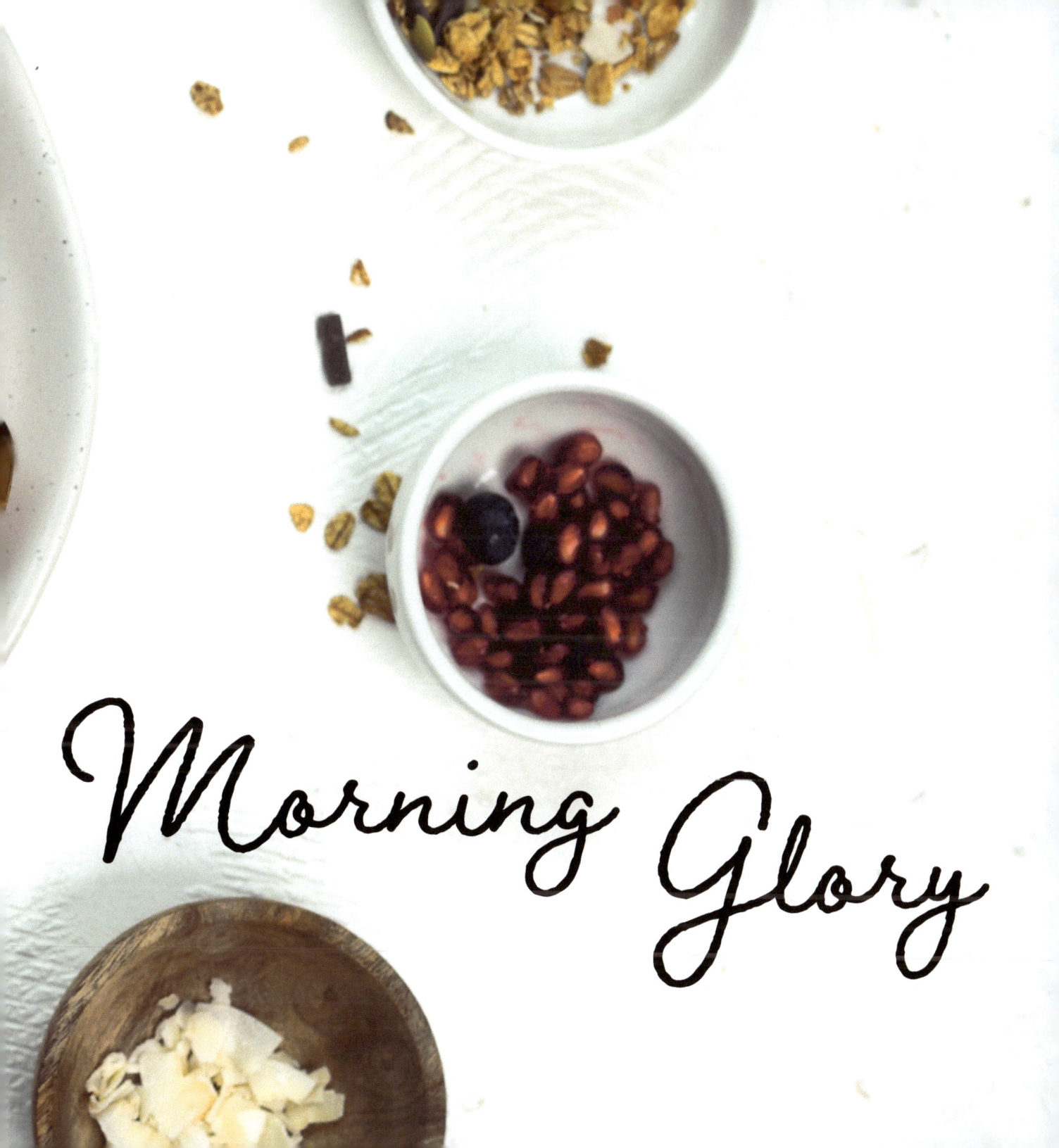

Morning Glory

Smoothies

Bananas are a good source of vitamins and minerals especially potassium and vitamin B6. A diet high in potassium benefits heart health.

Kale contains vitamins A, C, B and K and contains plant-based omega-3 fatty acids.

Berries are low in calories, high in fibre, vitamin C and antioxidants. Berries have proven benefits for heart health.

BANANA SMOOTHIE

150g whole almonds, soaked overnight, drained and rinsed

2 ripe bananas, peeled

1 tablespoon chia seeds

500ml water

GREEN SMOOTHIE

1 ripe banana, peeled

2 cups kale, washed and destemmed

2 tablespoons peanut butter

1 tablespoon soaked chia seeds

2 cups almond milk

2 dates

BERRY SMOOTHIE

1 banana

3 cups frozen berries of your choice

300ml almond milk or milk of your choice

125ml Greek yoghurt

Place all ingredients in a blender and process until smooth.

Pour into two glasses to serve.

If the smoothies are too thick add more milk or water to thin.

SERVES 2

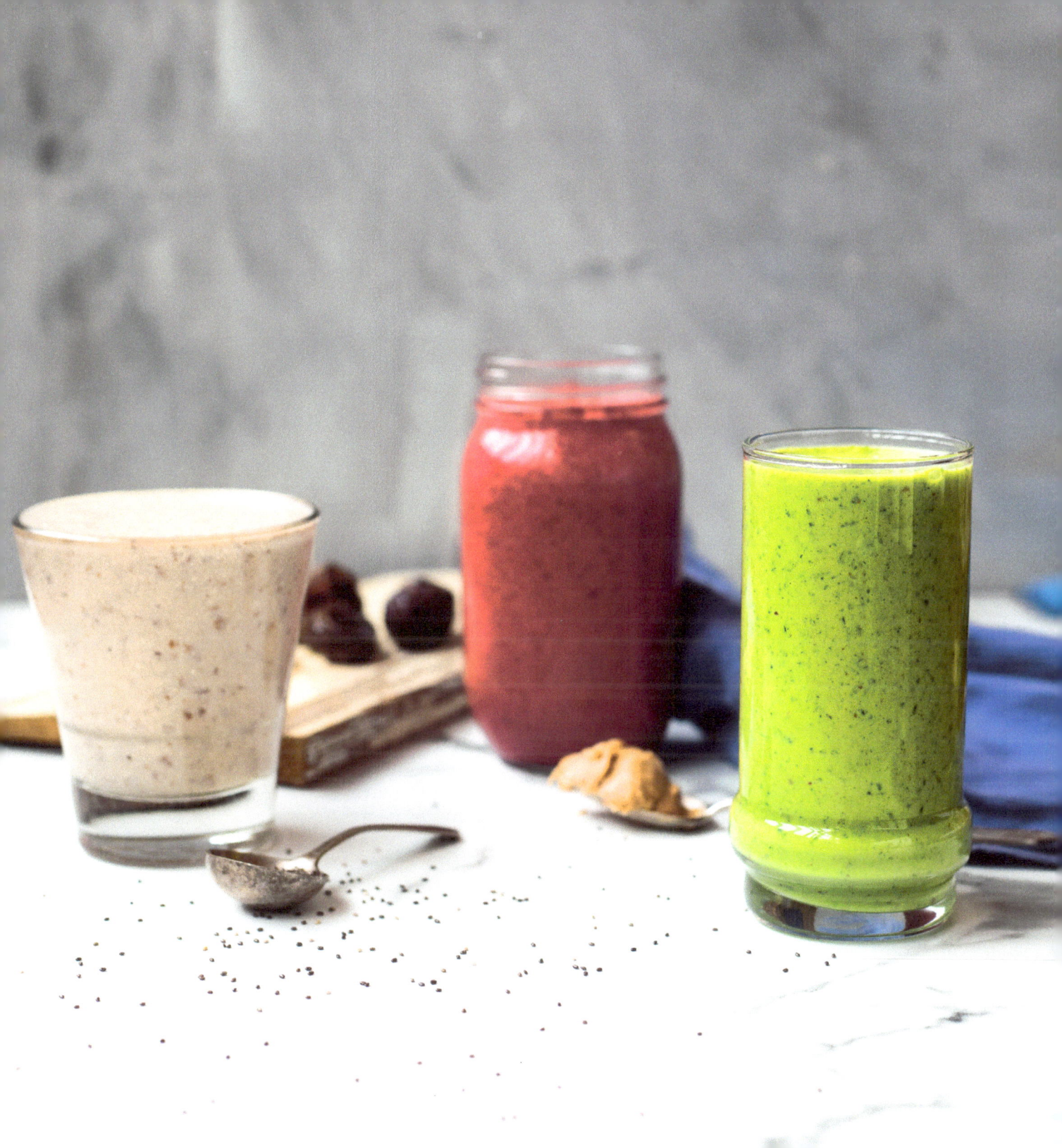

Overnight Oats

1 cup rolled oats
250ml almond milk
125ml Greek yoghurt
1 teaspoon vanilla extract
¼ teaspoon cinnamon
1 teaspoon chia seeds

Place all ingredients into a large glass container and mix until combined.

Put the top onto the container and place into the refrigerator overnight.

Eat with your favourite toppings the next day.

Overnight oats can be made up to five days ahead, refrigerated.

Add extra milk, if needed.

SERVES 2

Oats are a complex carbohydrate and a good source of fibre, manganese, iron, magnesium, zinc and selenium.

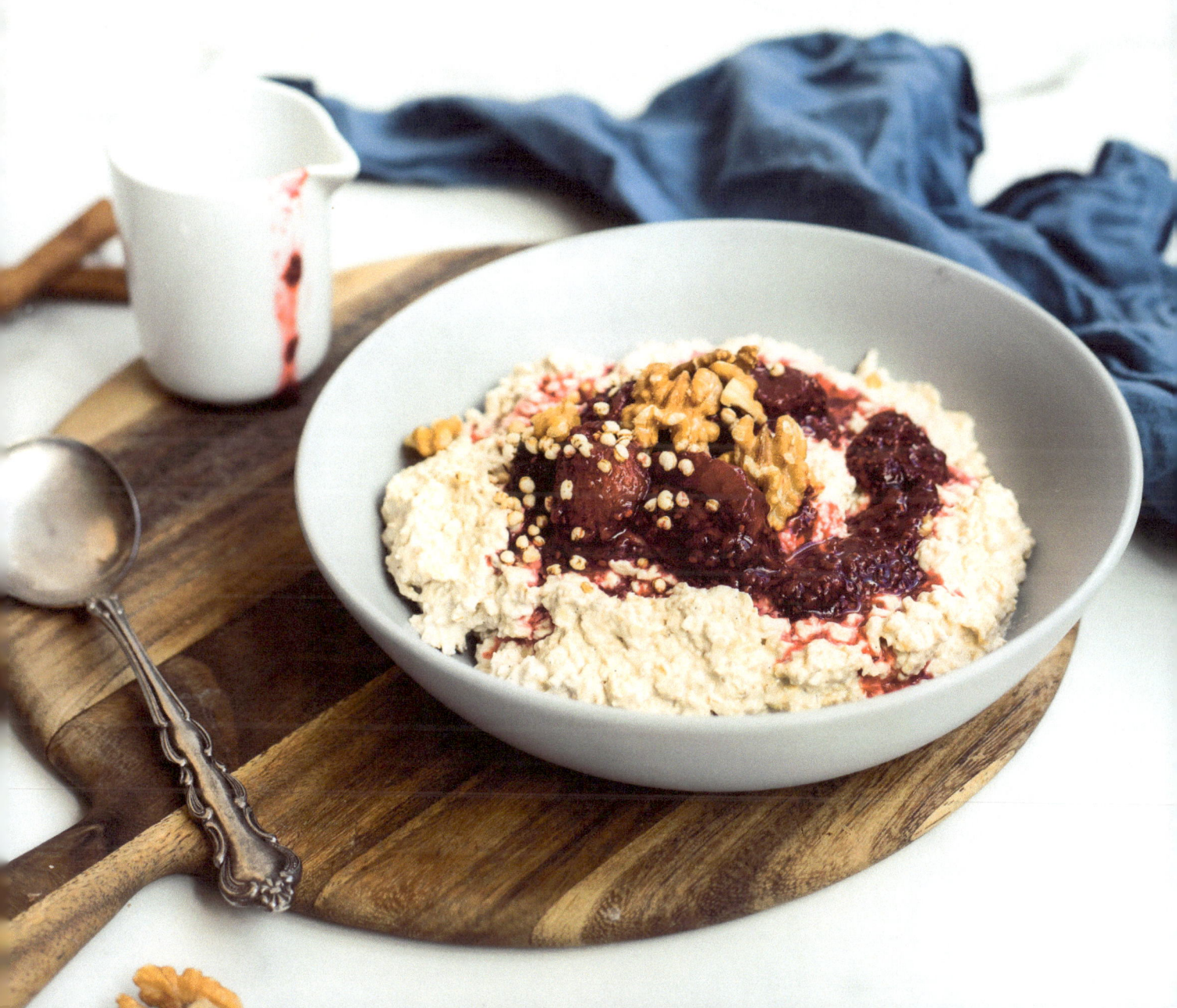

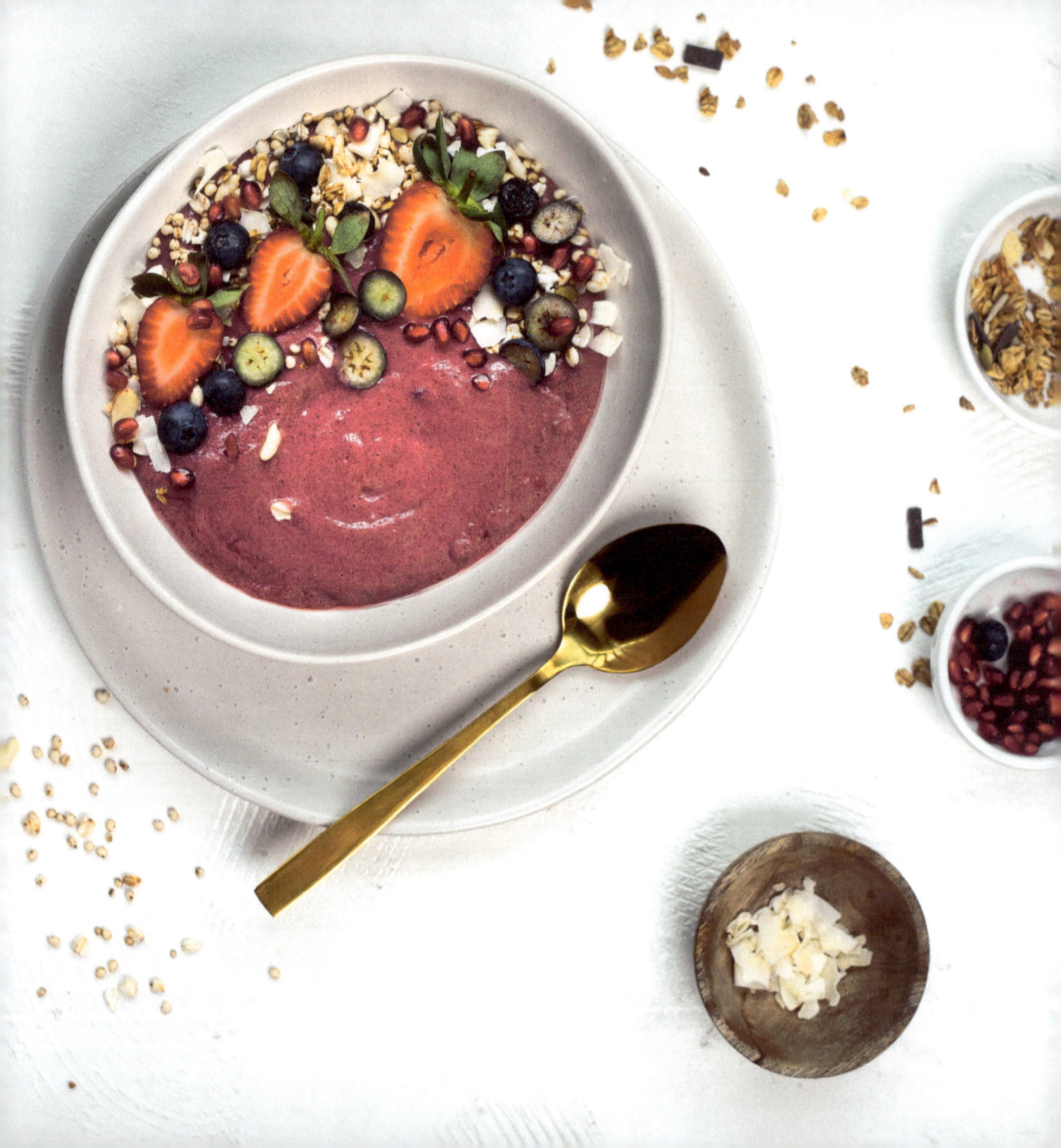

Acai Smoothie Bowl

400ml almond milk or milk of your choice

2 frozen bananas

2 medjool date

30g Organic Acai Smoothie Bowl packet or alternatively, 1 tablespoon of acai powder and one cup of berries

TOPPING SUGGESTIONS

Coconut flakes

Berries/fruit

Nuts

Puffed quinoa

Put all ingredients into a blender and blend until smooth.

Divide between two bowls and add toppings.

OPTIONAL: if you like your bowl a little sweeter add ½ to 1 teaspoon of maple syrup or honey and mix together prior to adding your toppings.

Blueberries are amongst the most nutrient-dense berries, are low in calories, high in fibre and antioxidants, and contain vitamins C and K and manganese.

SERVES 2

Chia Parfait

Chia seeds are high in plant-based omega-3 fatty acids, high in protein, contain fibre and antioxidants. Chia seeds are highly versatile as they absorb liquid and form a gel, they can be used as an egg replacement and used to thicken sauces.

4 tablespoons chia seeds

1 cup unsweetened almond milk

1/2 tablespoon maple syrup, honey or sweetener of choice

1/4 teaspoon vanilla

Toppings of choice: fresh berries, figs or other fruit, nuts etc.

In a bowl, stir together chia seeds, milk, maple syrup and vanilla.

Once the chia mixture is well combined, divide mixture into two glasses and cover. Put the glasses in the refrigerator and refrigerate overnight.

When ready to serve top with berries and/or your choice of fruit, yoghurt, nuts etc.

NOTE: chia parfait can be stored up to 5-7 days in the refrigerator.

SERVES 2

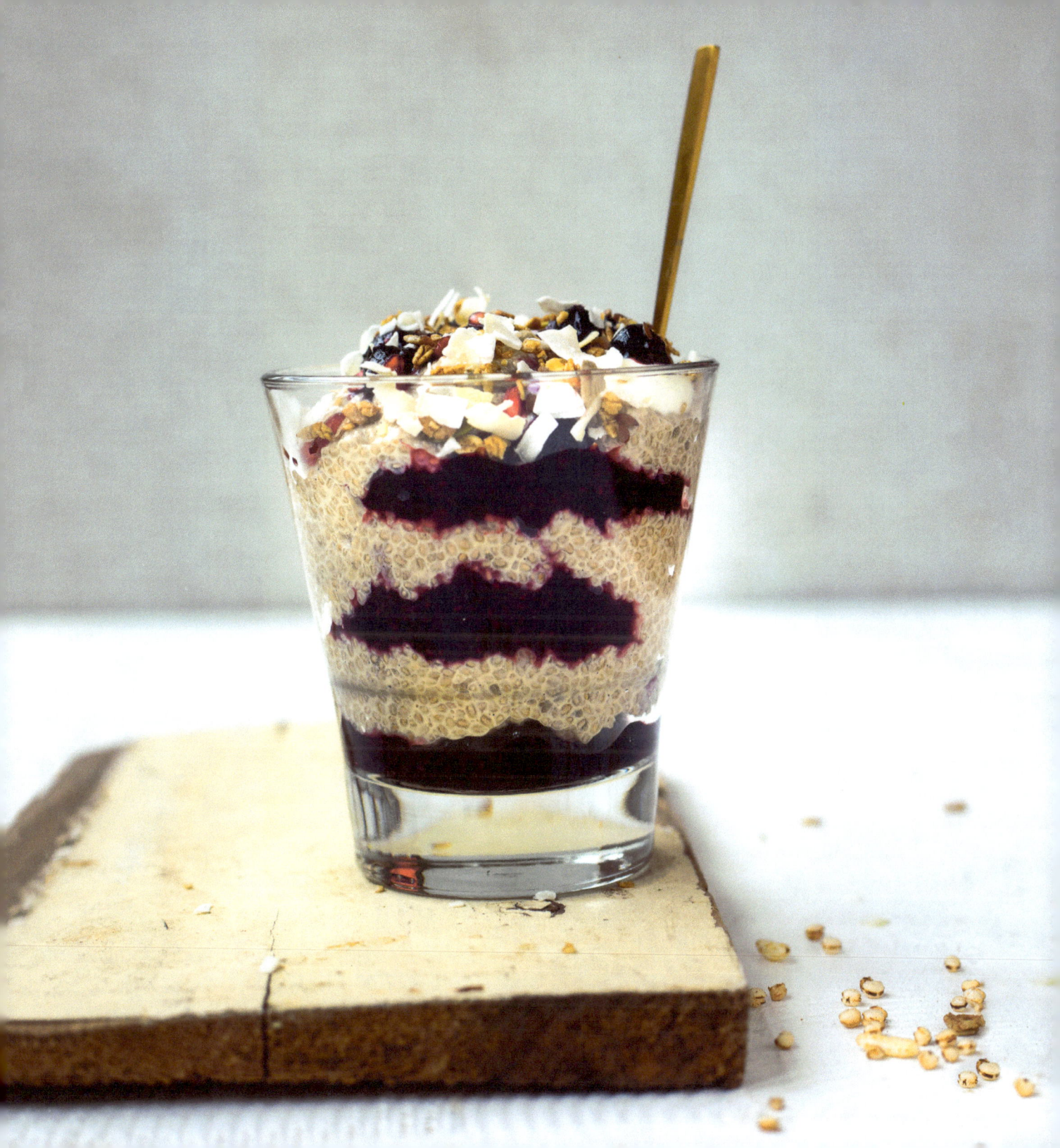

Starters / Light Lunch

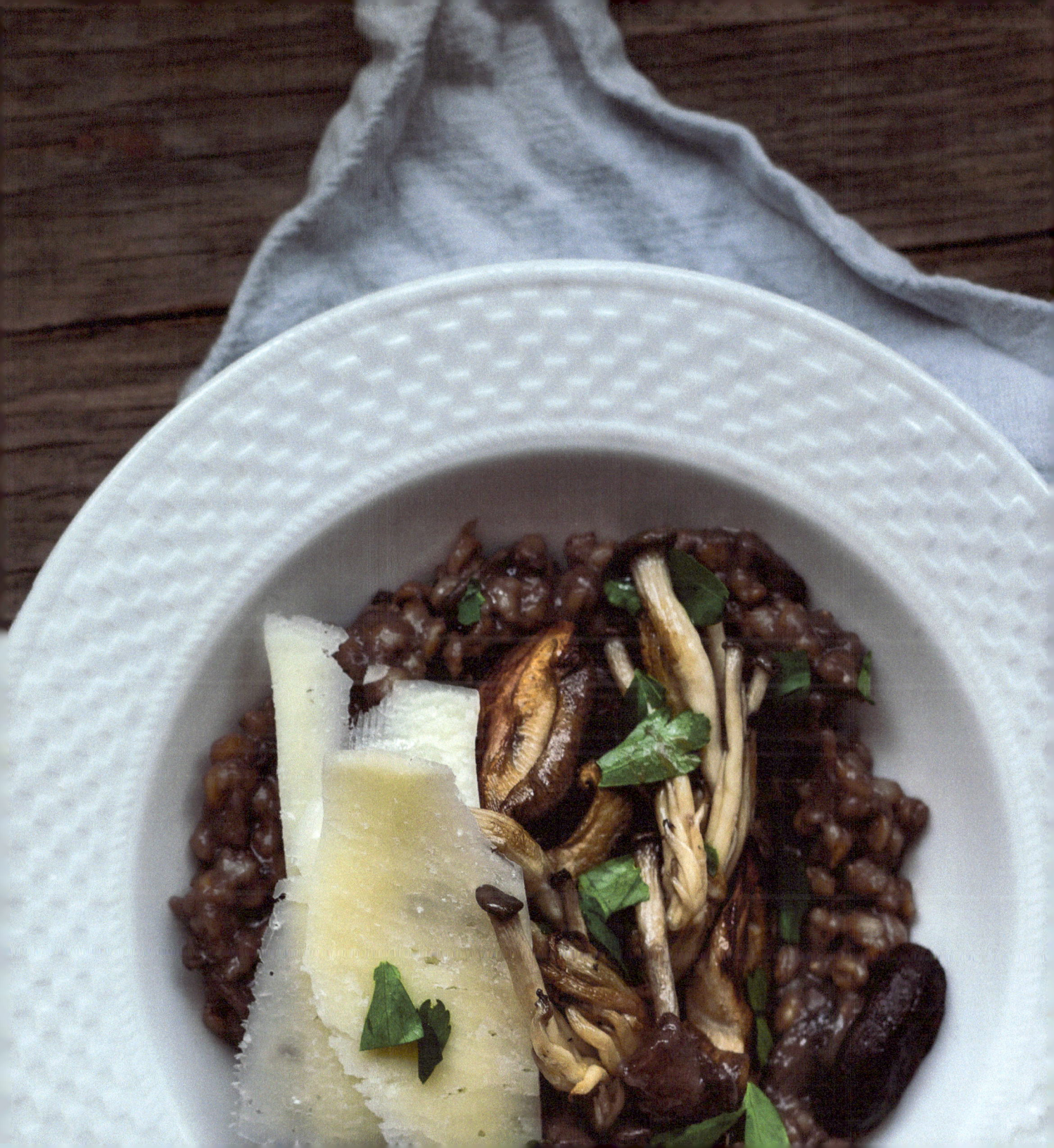

Tuna Salad on Seeded Crispbread

Although tuna is low in fat, tuna is still considered a good source of omega-3 fatty acids. Omega-3s are essential dietary fats that are beneficial for heart, eye and brain health.

425g can of tuna in brine
2 tablespoons mayonnaise
2 tablespoons Greek yoghurt
1 teaspoon horseradish mustard
100g of canned corn, drained
50g of cucumber, diced
½ red capsicum, seeds removed and diced
1 spring onion, sliced
Black pepper

SERVE WITH:
Microgreens
8 seeded crispbreads

Drain tuna and flake with the back of a fork. Place in a large bowl.

To the bowl of tuna, add the drained corn, diced cucumber, diced capsicum and sliced spring onion. Mix well to combine.

Place mayonnaise, yoghurt and horseradish mustard in a small bowl and mix well. Add mixture to the tuna bowl and combine.

Season with pepper.

TO SERVE: spoon onto seeded crispbreads and garnish with microgreens.

When entertaining, filling can be spooned onto small seeded crackers or fill some gem lettuce cups and serve.

Seeded crispbreads are readily available from your supermarket.

SERVES 4 FOR LIGHT LUNCH

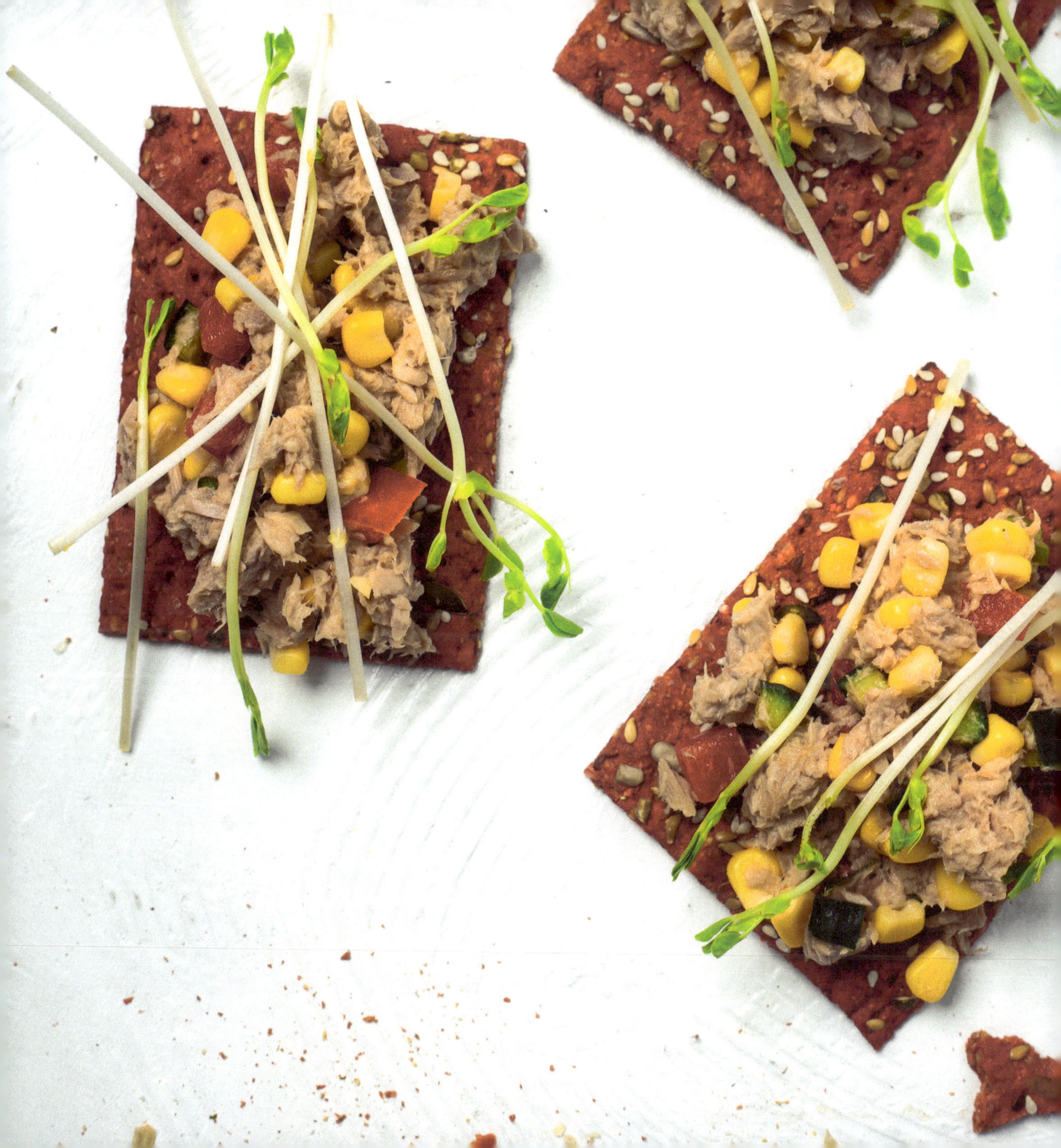

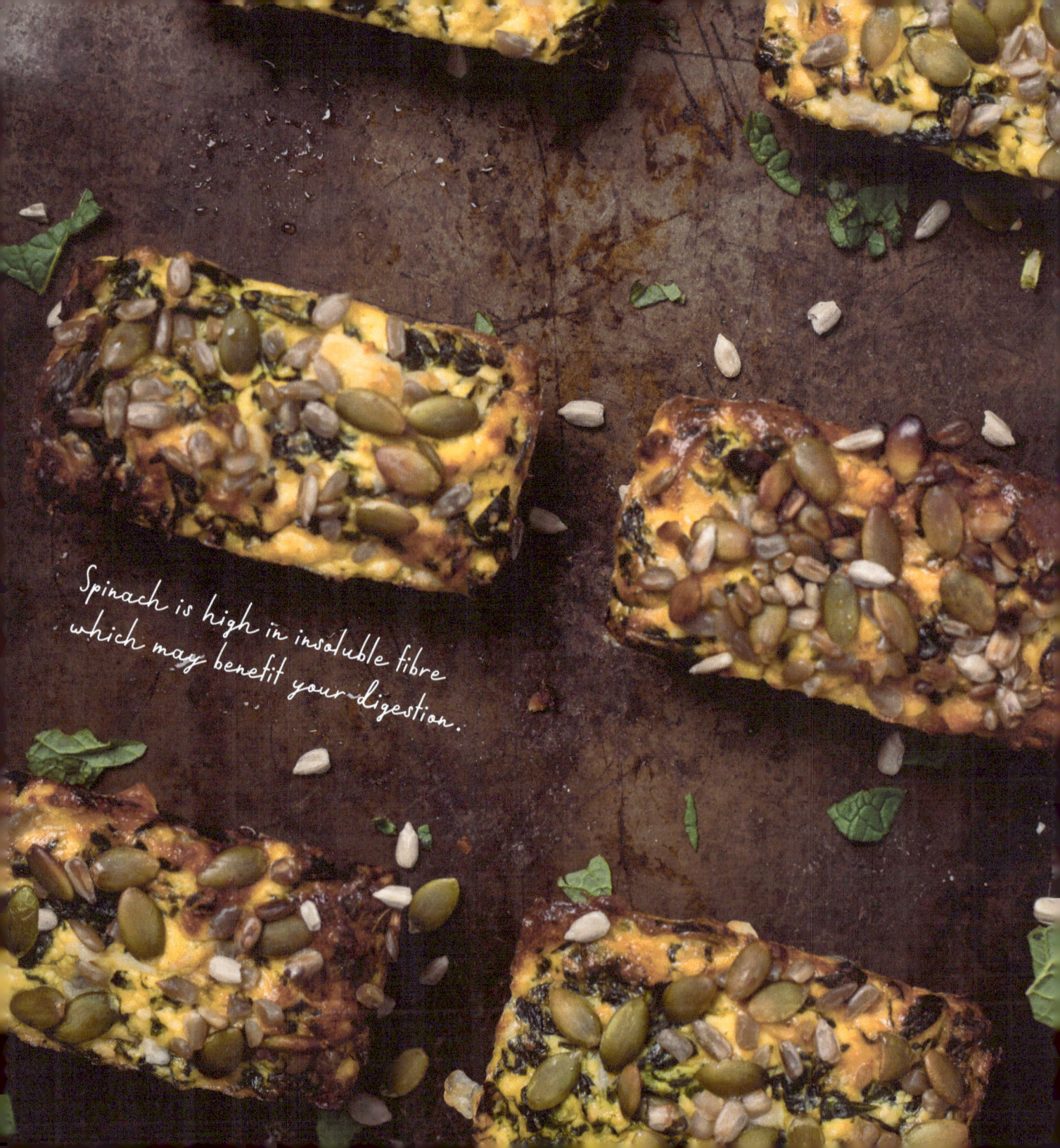

Spinach is high in insoluble fibre which may benefit your digestion.

Spinach and Ricotta Frittata

1 tablespoon light olive oil
250g ricotta cheese
125g grated parmesan cheese
3 eggs
125ml of yoghurt or sour cream
250g frozen spinach (thawed and drained well)
1 cup of mint leaves, chopped finely
1 tablespoon of sunflower seeds
1 tablespoon of pepita seeds

Preheat the oven to 180° Celsius.

Place the well drained spinach into a large bowl and stir in the mint.

In a separate large bowl, whisk the eggs. Add the ricotta cheese, yoghurt or sour cream and parmesan cheese to the eggs and mix to combine.

Place egg mixture into the spinach and mint and mix all the ingredients until you reach a smooth consistency.

Place contents into an oiled and lined cake pan, spreading mixture evenly.

Top with sunflower and pepita seeds.

Transfer to the oven and bake for 30 minutes.

Remove and rest for 5 minutes then turn out onto a plate.

Serve hot or cold.

NOTE: The frittata is suitable for freezing.

SERVES 6 FOR LIGHT LUNCH

Hot Smoked Salmon Salad

Salmon is rich in omega-3 fatty acids.

250g hot smoked salmon
250g cooked baby beetroot
2 tablespoons caperberries or capers
Oakleaf lettuce leaves
2 tablespoons crushed macadamia nuts
2 tablespoons mayonnaise
2 tablespoons yoghurt
1 teaspoon horseradish cream
1 teaspoon lemon juice
Dill sprigs, garnish

Cut beetroot into halves or quarters, depending on size.

Flake the hot smoked salmon into large pieces.

Put the mayonnaise, yoghurt and horseradish cream into a bowl and whisk to combine. Add lemon juice. Season with salt and pepper and mix through thoroughly. Add a little water if mixture is too thick.

Divide lettuce between two plates, top with beetroot, salmon, caperberries or capers.

Drizzle over mayonnaise dressing and garnish with dill and nuts.

SERVES 2 FOR LIGHT LUNCH

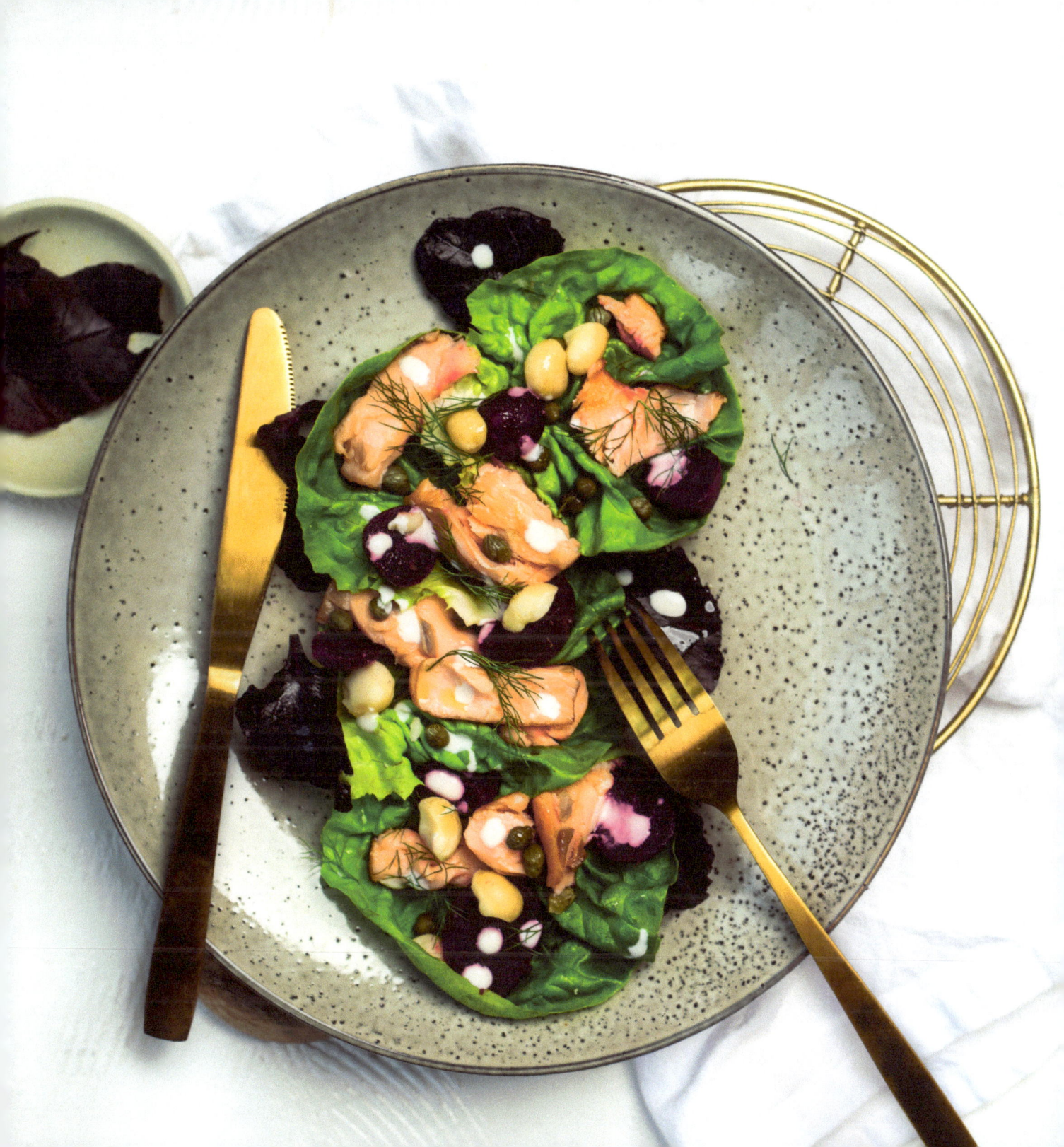

Mushroom Barley Risotto

The glycaemic load of mushrooms is very low, they have a very small amount of fat, provide a small amount of protein and they are full of nutrients. Mushrooms can be very beneficial to one's health and wellbeing.

- 3 tablespoons olive oil
- 500g field mushrooms
- 10g dried porcini mushrooms
- 200g of exotic mushrooms
- 1 onion
- 2 cloves of garlic
- 250ml red dry wine
- 5 cups of beef stock
- 200g pearl barley
- 2 teaspoons dijon mustard
- 50g parmesan cheese, shaved

Place the porcini in a bowl of water and soak for 10 minutes.

Heat 2 tablespoons of oil in a frypan over high heat. Add field and exotic mushrooms and cook, stirring for 3-5 minutes. Remove from pan and set aside.

Return pan to medium heat and add oil. Add onion, cook until softened. Add the garlic, drained porcini, mustard, barley and thyme and cook for a further 2 minutes or until fragrant. Add the wine, stock and bring to a simmer.

Reduce heat to medium low and cook stirring occasionally until liquid is absorbed and the barley is tender. Approximately 40 minutes.

To SERVE: top with reserved mushrooms and parmesan cheese.

SERVES 4

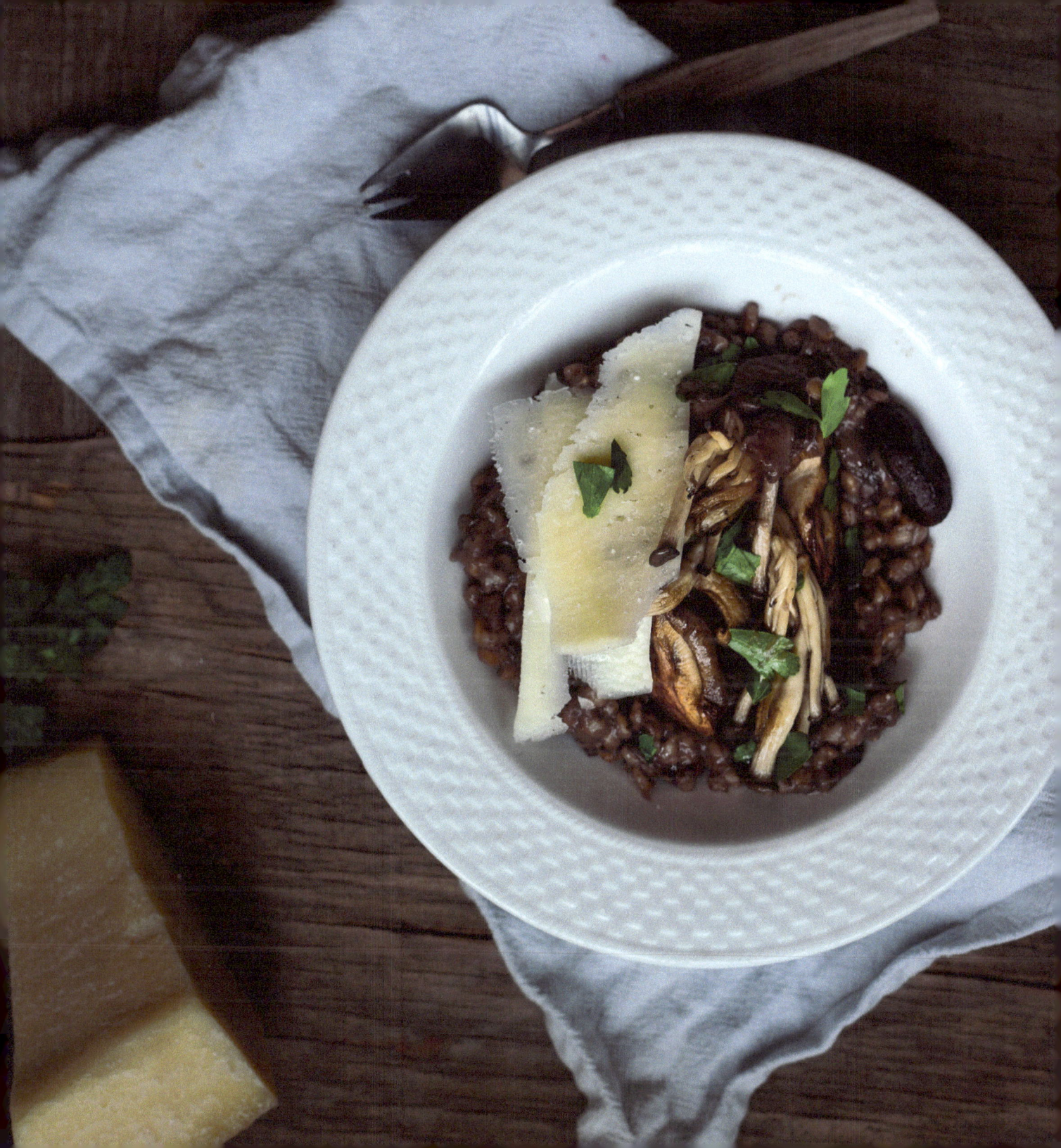

Sharing Plates

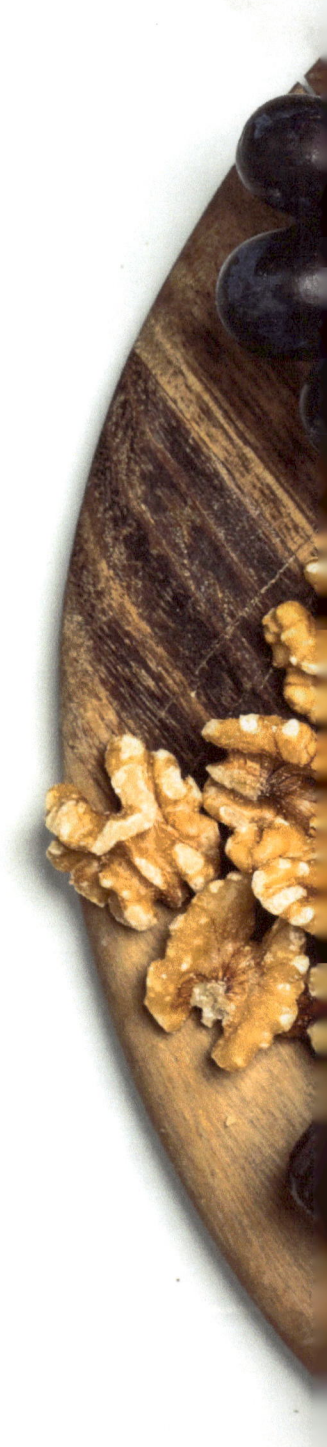

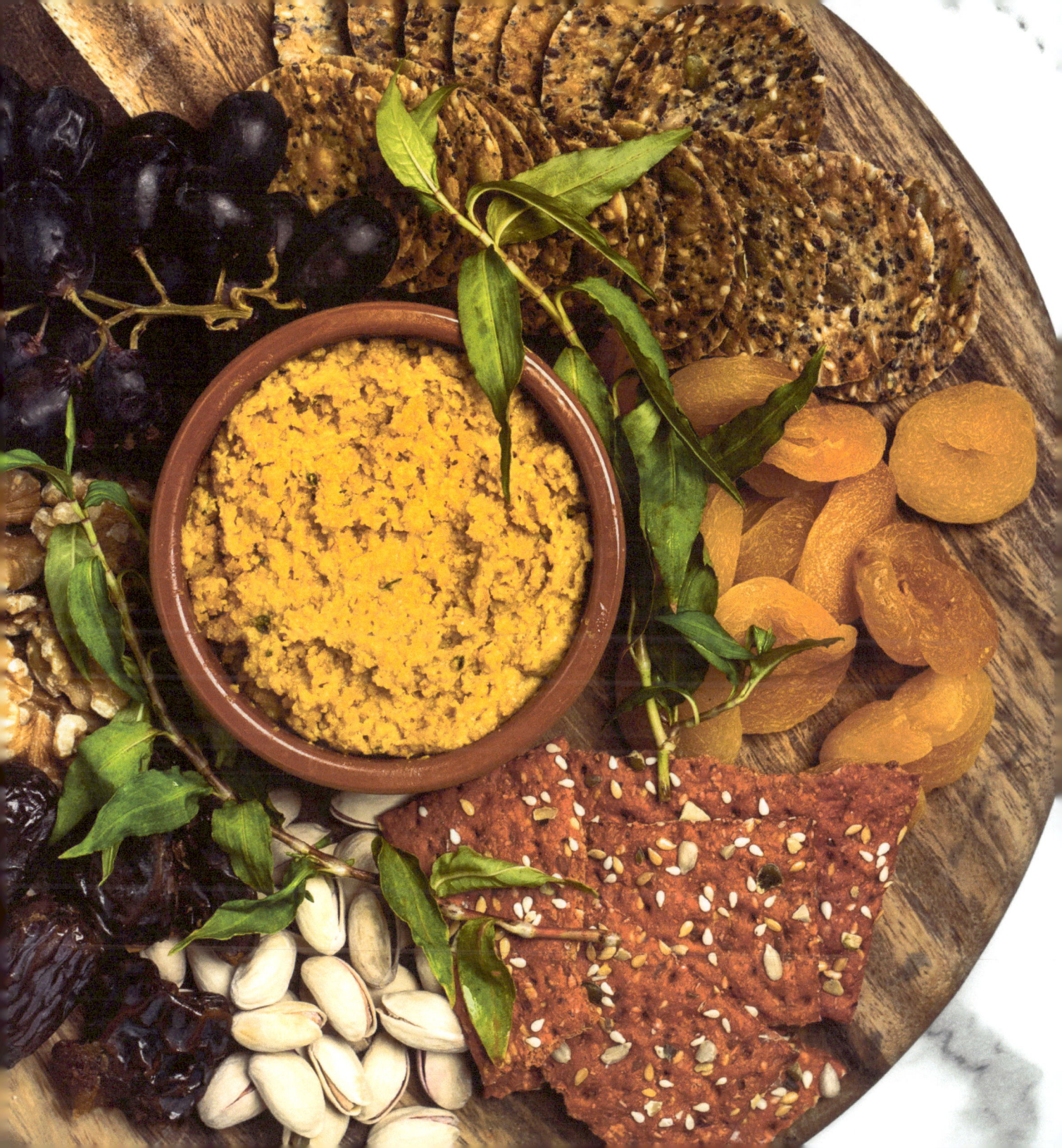

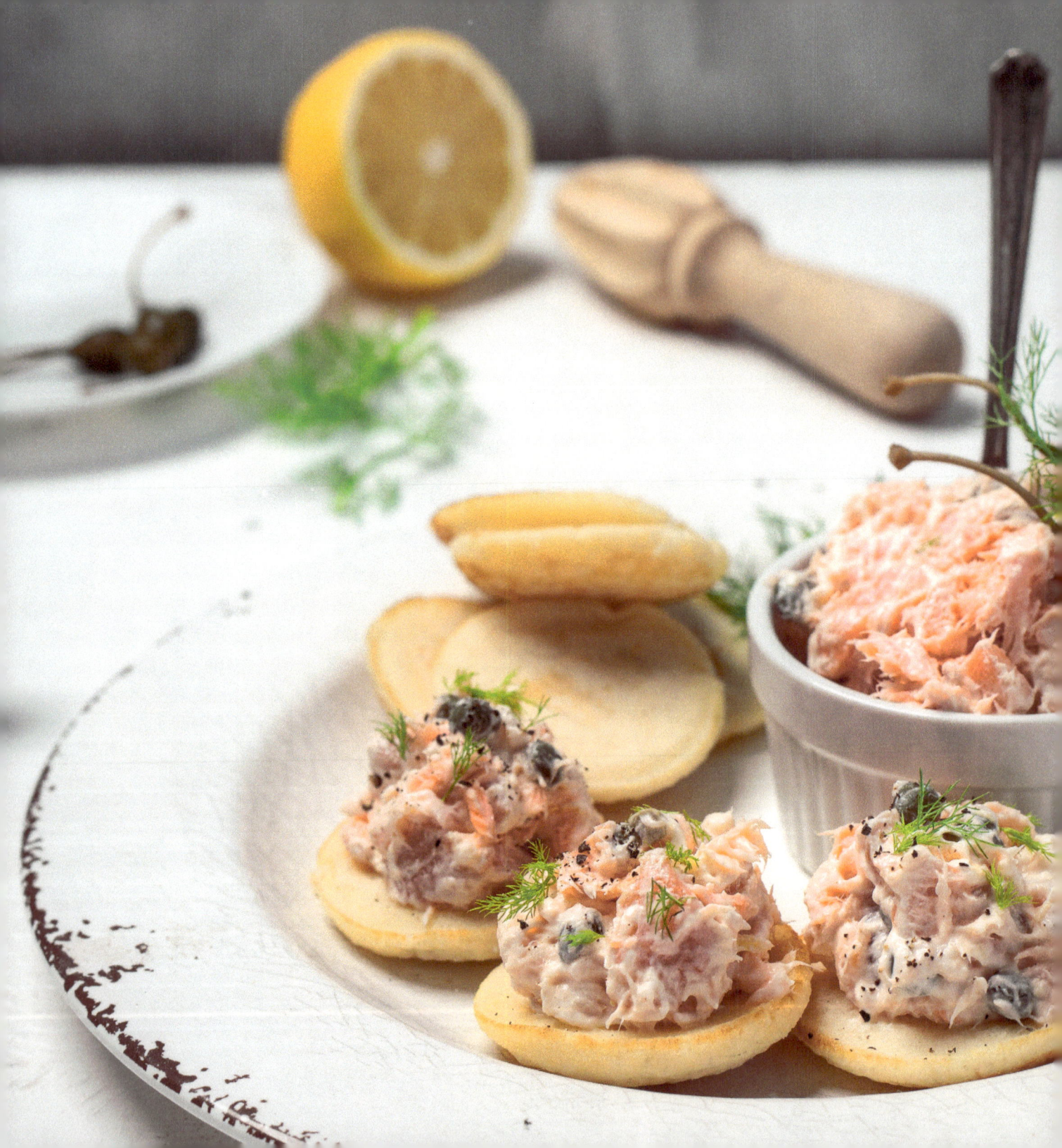

Hot and Cold Salmon Pâté

Capers contain Vitamins A and E and play a role in limiting oxidative stress.

250g hot smoked salmon
250g smoked salmon
120g sour cream
2 tsp horseradish cream
2 tsp capers, chopped
Juice and zest of 1 lemon
2 sprigs dill chopped
Black pepper

TO SERVE
Blini or seeded crackers

Finely chop the smoked salmon and place in a bowl with the sour cream, capers, and horseradish, lemon juice and zest.

Season with a little pepper and fold the ingredients together.

Flake the hot smoked salmon and gently fold into the cream mixture taking care not to over work the pâté.

Place in the refrigerator to chill.

Once chilled serve on blini or seeded crackers.

SERVES 4

Chicken Larb on Lettuce Cups

1 tablespoon peanut oil

500g lean minced chicken

1 garlic clove minced

1 large red chilli, finely sliced

2 teaspoons fresh ginger minced

1 teaspoon turmeric

1 onion finely diced

2 lemongrass stalks, finely minced

4 spring onions, sliced

2 tablespoons fish sauce,

5 tablespoon lime juice

½ bunch coriander, leaves and stems chopped

½ bunch Vietnamese mint, leaves chopped

½ bunch basil leaves, leaves chopped

5 kaffir lime leaves, finely chopped, discard vein

½ bunch fresh mint, leaves chopped

Baby gem lettuce leaves

Crushed peanuts, garnish

Wash the lettuce leaves and dry thoroughly.

Heat oil in a pan over low heat, add ginger, turmeric and chilli and stir to release the aromas. Add the onion, garlic, lemongrass and spring onions and saute until softened.

Increase the heat and add the chicken and cook, until the chicken is cooked thoroughly. Breaking up lumps as you go.

Stir in the fish sauce, add the lime juice and herbs and combine well. Turn off heat.

TO SERVE: fill lettuce cups with one or two tablespoons of chicken mixture, depending on the size of your lettuce cups and garnish with crushed peanuts.

Herbs are a fantastic way to add flavour and colour to your meal, without adding fat, salt or sugar. Herbs also tend to have their own set of health-promoting properties.

SERVES 4

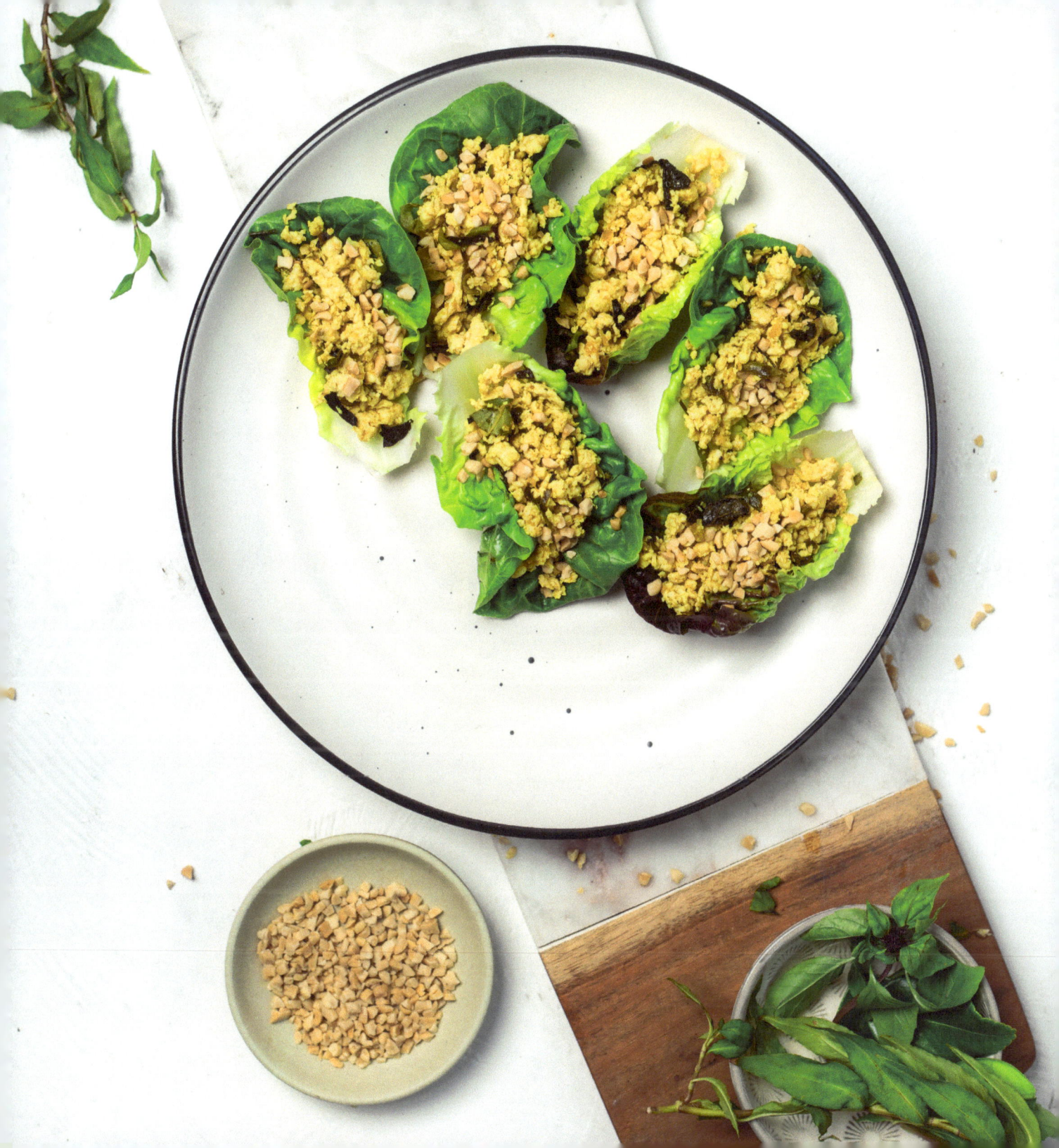

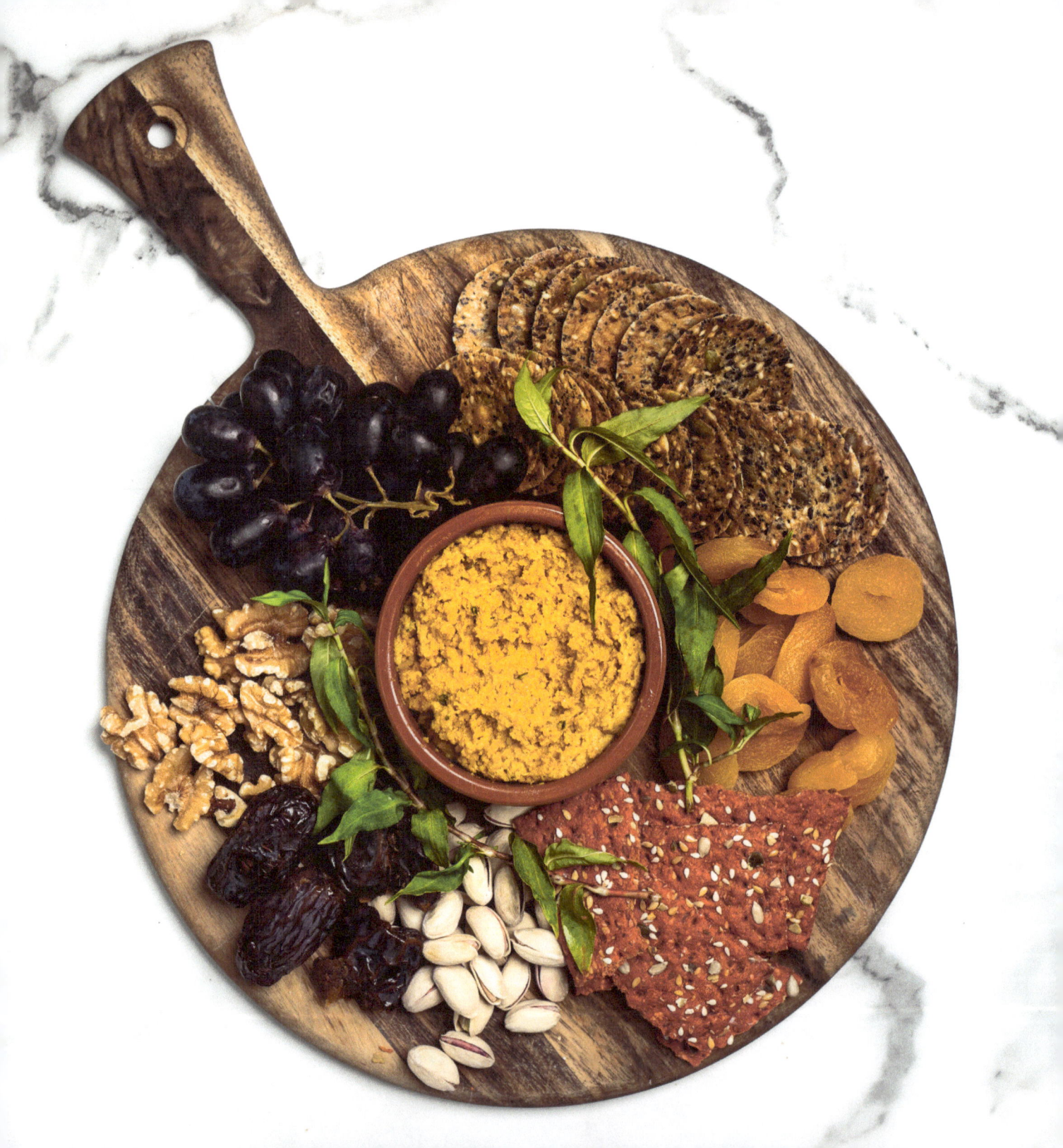

Nut Cheese Platter

Cashews are rich in unsaturated fats. They contain protein, fibre, copper, magnesium, manganese and are low in sugar.

1 cup cashew nuts
2 tablespoons nutritional yeast
1/4 teaspoon sea salt flakes
¼ teaspoon white pepper
¼ teaspoon garlic powder
1 teaspoon turmeric
2 tablespoons lemon juice
1 teaspoon picked thyme
1 teaspoon dried rosemary

Soak the cashew nuts overnight.

Drain and rinse the nuts well.

Process nuts in a blender, stopping to scrape down the sides occasionally.

Add remaining ingredients and process until well combined.

If necessary, adjust with a little water.

Transfer to a bowl and serve.

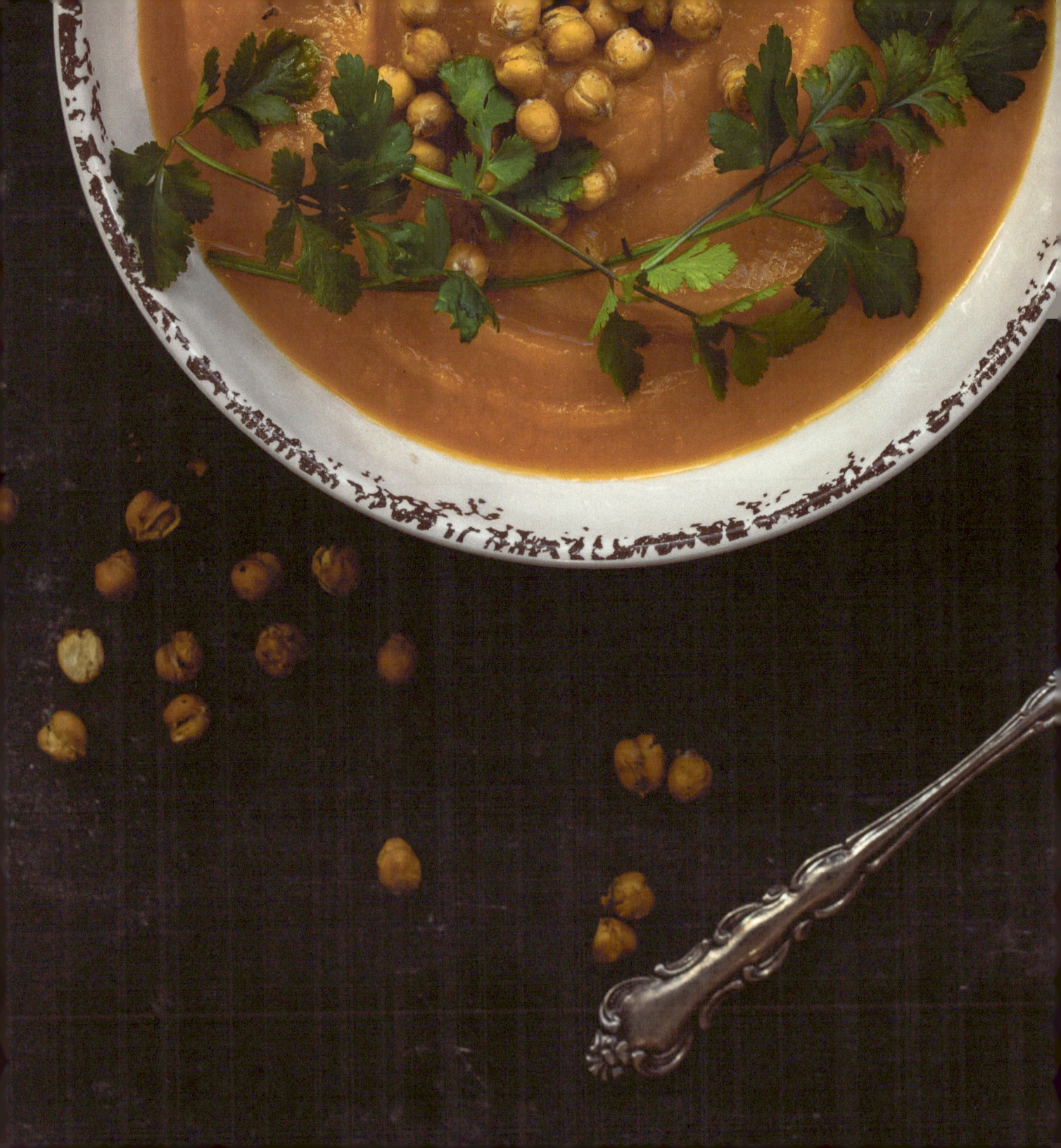

Nourishing Bowls

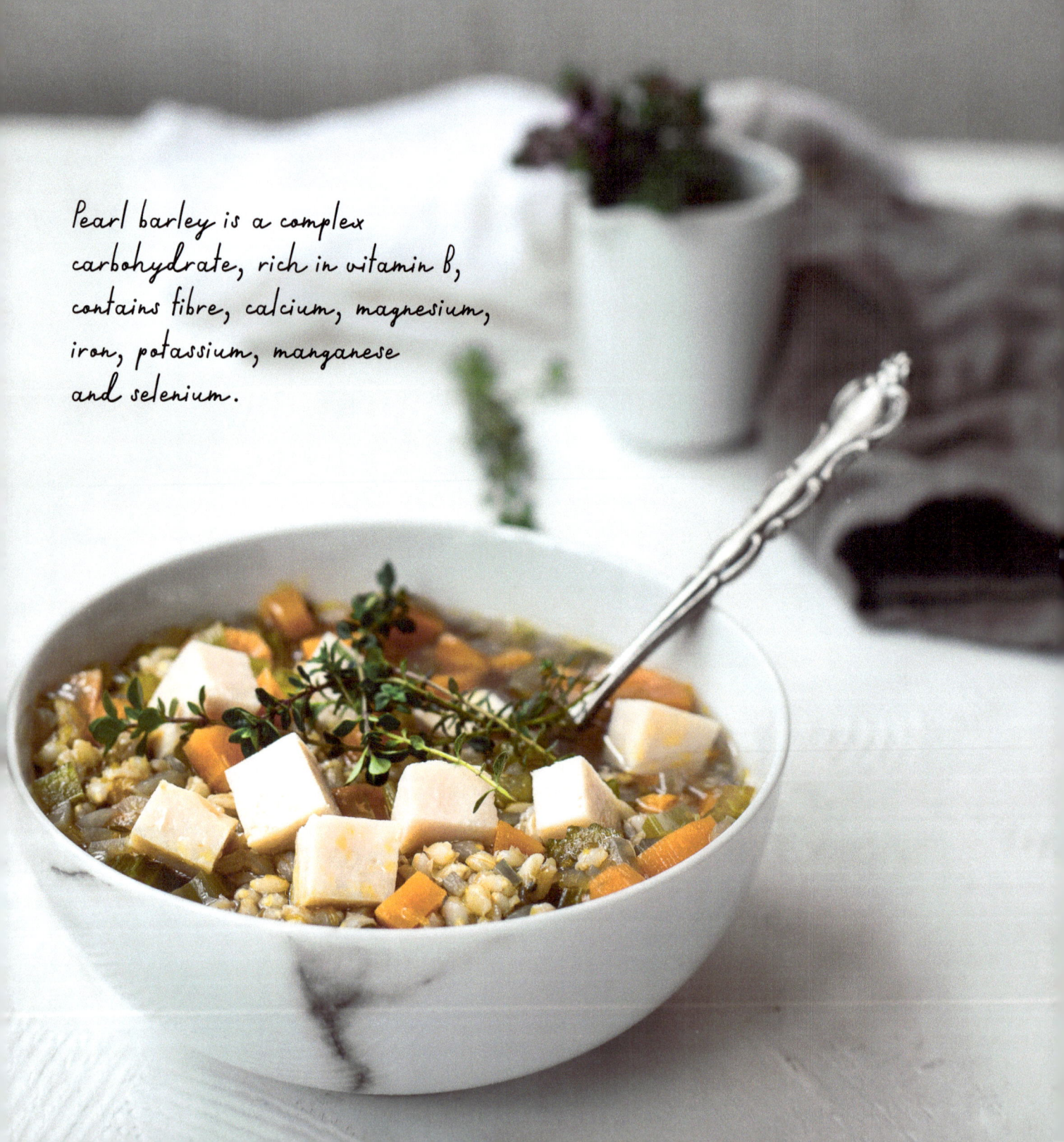

Pearl barley is a complex carbohydrate, rich in vitamin B, contains fibre, calcium, magnesium, iron, potassium, manganese and selenium.

Soffrito Bowl with Barley and Smoked Chicken

1 tablespoon oil

1 onion

3 carrots

2 sticks celery

1 bunch of fresh lemon thyme leaves, picked

600ml stock (chicken or vegetable)

300g smoked chicken, chopped

1 cup cooked barley

Peel and dice the onions and carrots. Dice the celery. Place the oil in a pot and sweat the onion, carrot and celery in oil until softened.

Add half the thyme leaves.

Add the stock and bring to a gentle simmer.

Add the cooked barley, smoked chicken and additional thyme and simmer for another 5 minutes before serving.

ALTERNATIVE: interchange smoked chicken for cooked chicken breast or turkey breast.

Barley can be interchanged with a grain of your choice, quinoa, freekeh or brown rice.

SERVES 2

Quick Chicken Pho

1 litre chicken stock
Bunch coriander chopped roughly
Vietnamese mint, leaves picked
Thai basil, leaves picked
1 long red chilli, sliced
2cm ginger, julienned
2 medium spring onions, sliced
2 teaspoons coriander seeds
1 whole star anise
1 cinnamon stick
1 black cardamon pod, crushed
1 garlic clove
200g chicken breast
100g soba noodles
3 teaspoons fish sauce
2 limes, cut into wedges

Place coriander seeds into a dry hot pan and toast for a few minutes or until aromatic. Add the ginger and stir for one minute.

Place stock in a large pot over medium heat.

Add the coriander seeds, ginger, star anise, cardamon, garlic, spring onions and cinnamon stick into the stock.

Bring the stock to the boil and simmer for 15 minutes.

Add your chicken breast and poach for 10 minutes. Remove the chicken and cut into slices.

Continue simmering the stock for another 5 minutes.

Cook noodles according to the packet instructions.

Strain the noodles from the water. Divide the noodles amongst four bowls and top with chicken.

Season the stock with fish sauce.

Ladle stock into each bowl and garnish with coriander, Vietnamese mint, Thai basil, chilli, and lime wedges.

SERVES 4

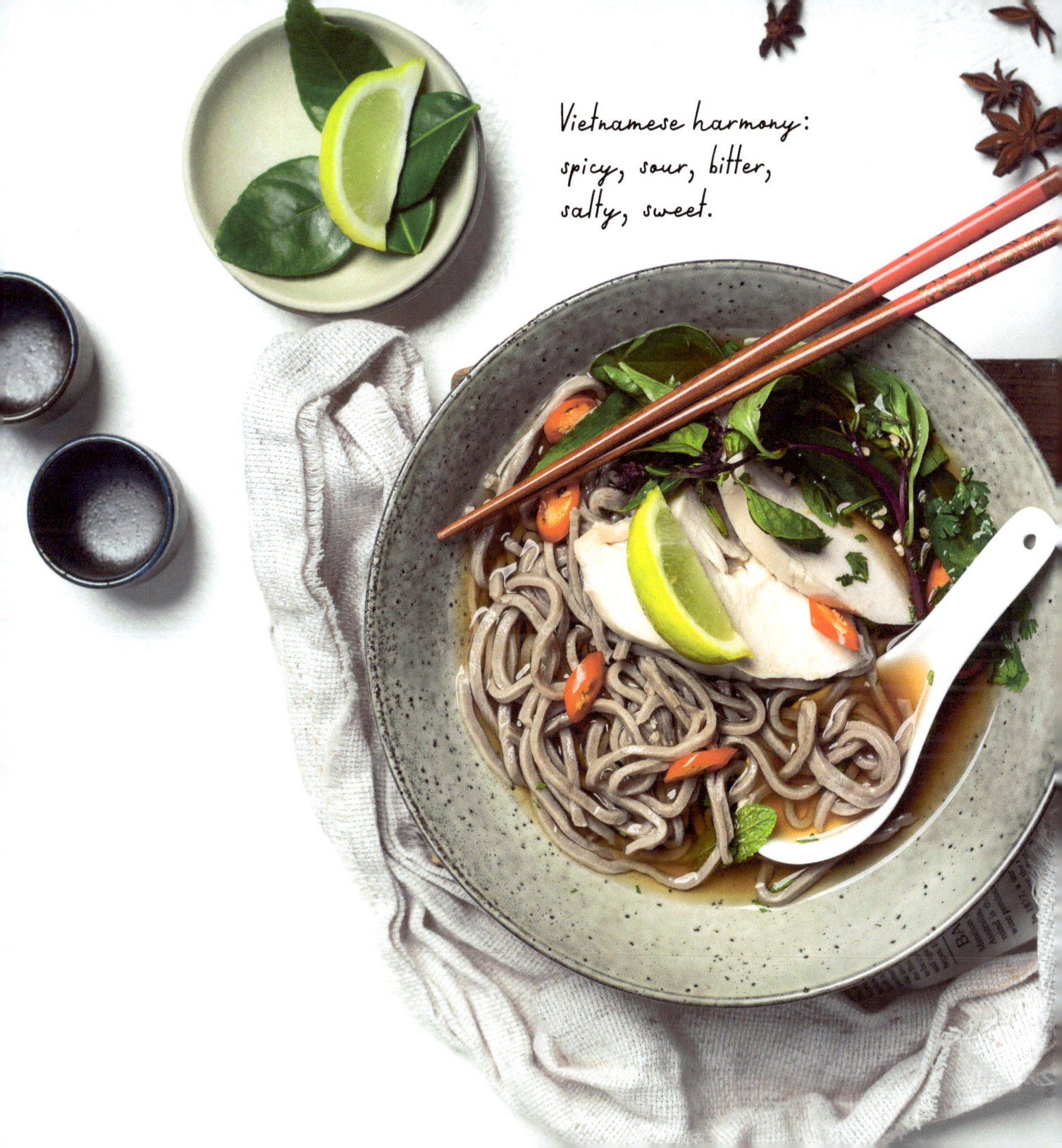

Vietnamese harmony: spicy, sour, bitter, salty, sweet.

Pumpkin Soup with Spiced Chickpeas

CHICKPEAS

2 teaspoons coconut oil

400g tinned chickpeas, drained and rinsed

¾ teaspoon sea salt flakes

½ teaspoon freshly ground black pepper

1 teaspoon dried oregano

1 teaspoon dried rosemary

¼ teaspoon cayenne pepper

PUMPKIN SOUP

1 kg pumpkin chopped

2 cups chopped carrots

2 medium sweet potatoes

1 onion diced

5g pepper

Salt

Bay leaf

1.5 litres water

CHICKPEAS

Preheat oven to 180° Celsius.

Spoon the coconut oil into a small pan and warm in the oven for 1-2 minutes until melted.

Pat the drained, rinsed chickpeas with kitchen paper and discard any of the loose skins.

In a bowl, mix all the remaining ingredients and chickpeas together with the coconut oil until well combined. Make sure the chickpeas are evenly coated.

Place onto a baking tray and bake for 30-35 minutes. The chickpeas are ready when they are a golden-brown colour and have a little crunch to them.

PUMPKIN SOUP

Add the pumpkin, sweet potato, carrots, onion, bay leaves, water and simmer for 1 hour or until pumpkin is soft. Blend soup until smooth with stick blender.

Season to taste.

TO SERVE: add spiced baked chickpeas on top of pumpkin soup

NOTE: chickpeas can be eaten on their own as a healthy snack.

SERVES 4

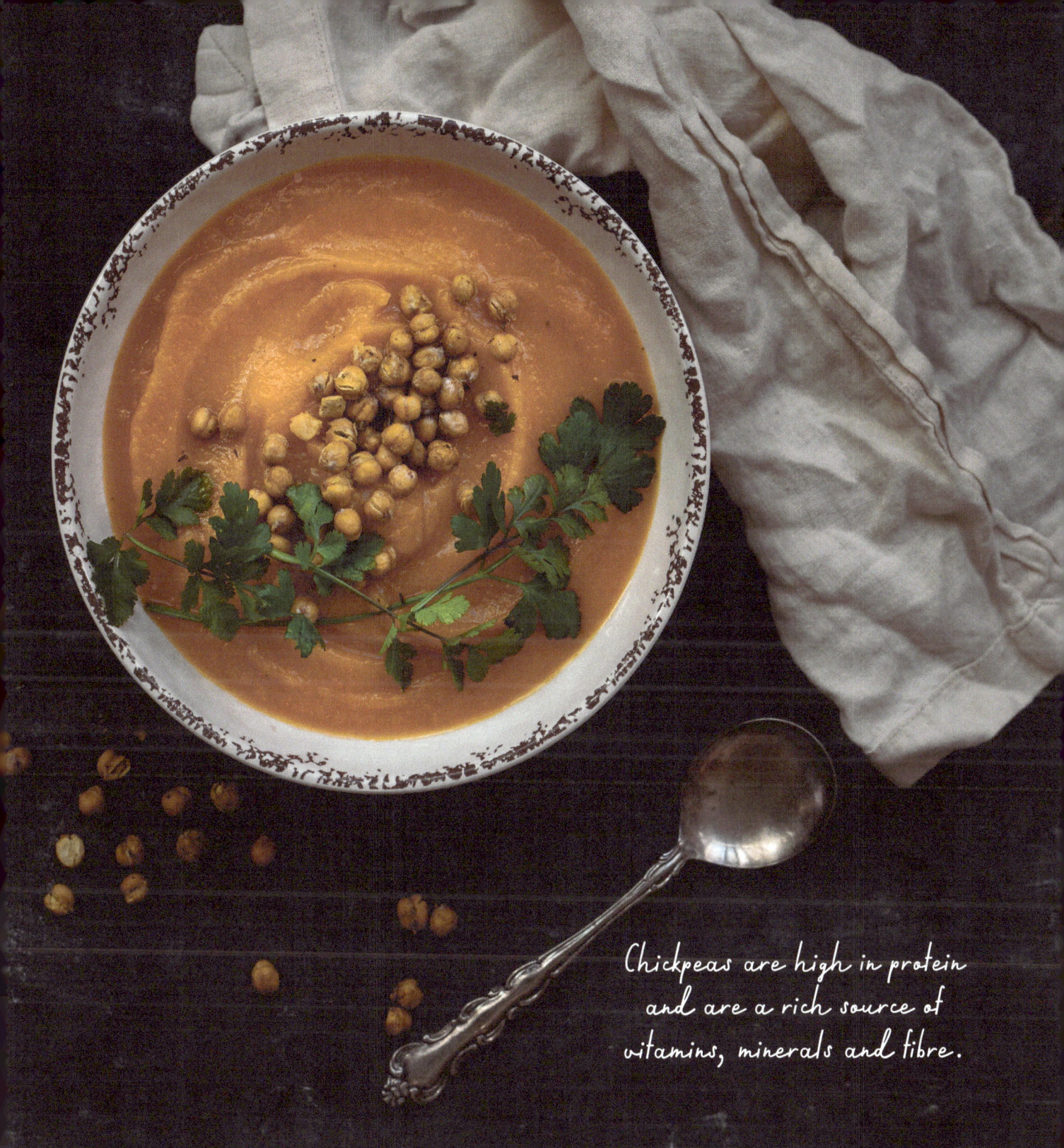

Chickpeas are high in protein and are a rich source of vitamins, minerals and fibre.

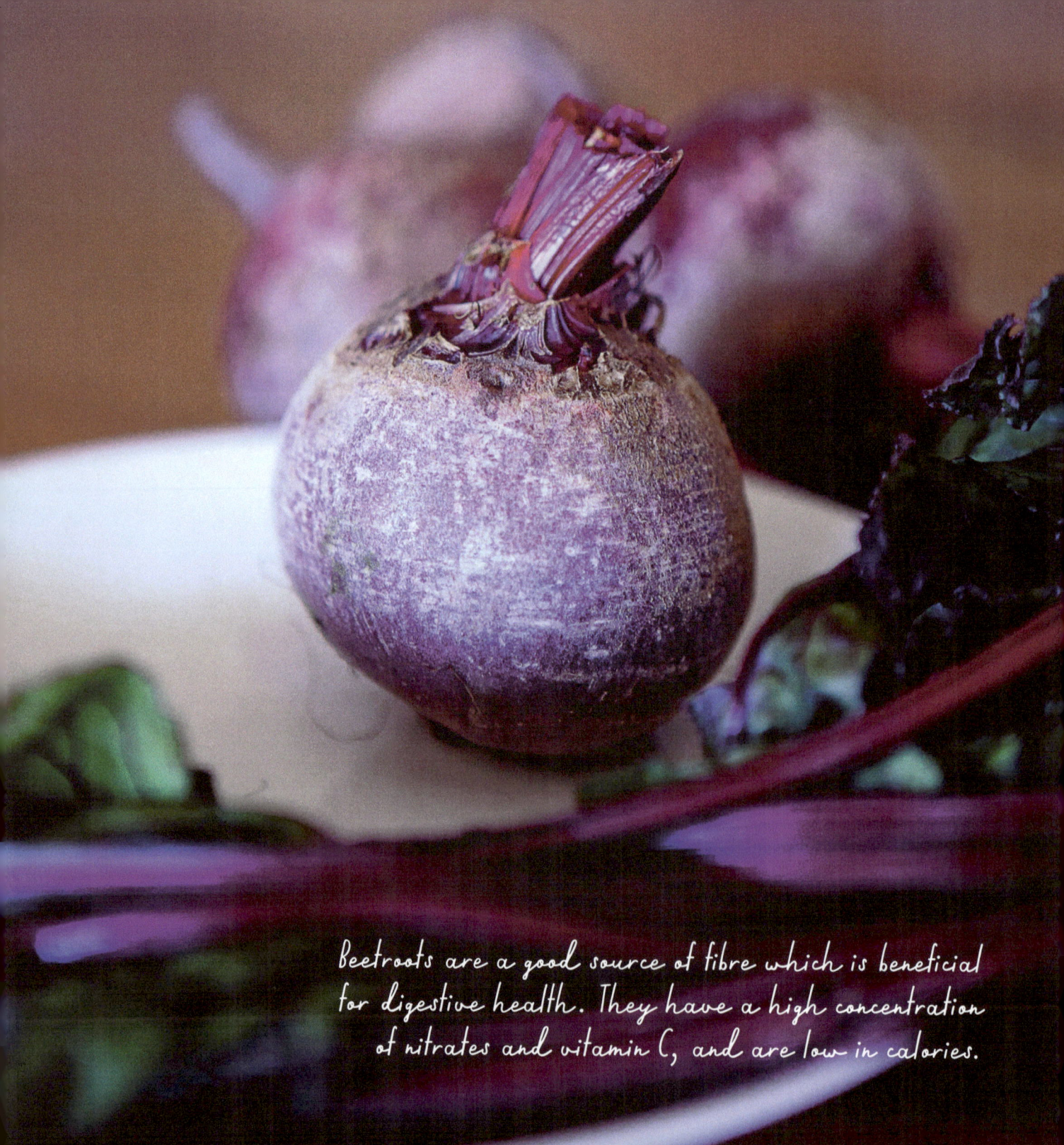

Beetroots are a good source of fibre which is beneficial for digestive health. They have a high concentration of nitrates and vitamin C, and are low in calories.

Beetroot and Orange Cured Salmon

1 x 250g salmon fillet, middle cut, skinned and pin boned

1 tablespoons sea salt

1 teaspoon fennel seeds

2 tablespoons pomegranate molasses

150g raw beetroot, grated

zest from 1 orange

Small bunch of dill, chopped

Combine all the ingredients together in a bowl, except the salmon.

Lay out 3 layers of clingwrap on a board. Place salmon on the clingwrap and press the mixture onto the salmon fillet. Wrap the fillet and mixture tightly in the cling wrap and place in a bowl and weigh down with a heavy item on top.

Chill for a minimum of 48 hours but preferably 72 hours.

Once ready, unwrap the salmon and discard the mixture.

Rinse under cold running water, pat dry with kitchen paper and wrap in fresh clingwrap. Keep chilled until ready to serve.

Salmon will keep refrigerated for 3 to 5 days

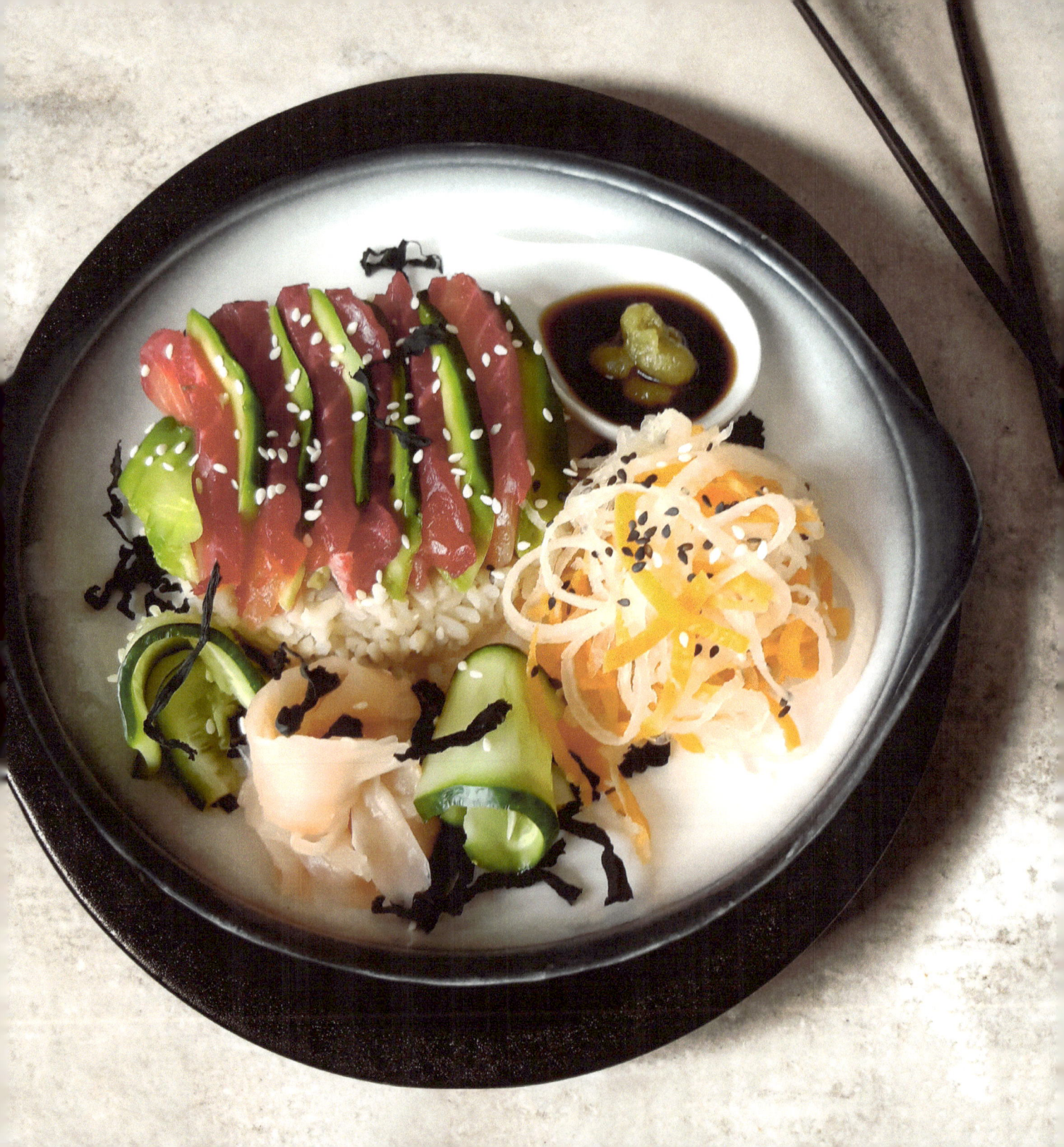

Cured Salmon Poke Bowl

Brown rice is highly nutritious providing a wide range of vitamins, minerals and antioxidants.

Beetroot and Orange Cured Salmon, see recipe on page 73
1 avocado
4 cups cooked brown rice
30g sushi rice seasoning
80g pickled ginger and juice
Small daikon, shredded
1 large carrot, shredded
1 cucumber cut into ribbons
2 teaspoons wasabi
4 tablespoons soy sauce

GARNISH
Sesame seeds black and white
Dried sliced seaweed

Slice cured salmon very finely.

Cut avocado in half and cut into slices.

Combine brown rice with some pickling juice and sushi rice seasoning.

Divide the rice between four bowls.

Place avocado slices and cured salmon on top of rice.

Arrange daikon and carrot on plate along with cucumber ribbons and pickled ginger.

Place soy sauce in a small bowl and add ½ teaspoon wasabi.

Garnish with sesame seeds and dried seaweed.

ALTERNATIVE: replace cured salmon for sashimi grade fish of your liking, smoked trout or tinned tuna or salmon.

SERVES 4

Vietnamese Cabbage and Poached Chicken Salad

Vietnamese mint contains good chemicals called flavonoids. These flavonoids work as antioxidants.

2 boneless skinless chicken breasts
½ cabbage, shredded
2 carrots, julienned
2 spring onions, finely sliced
1 long red chilli, sliced
½ bunch Vietnamese mint, leaves chopped
½ bunch mint leaves, chopped
½ bunch coriander, leaves and stems chopped
4 tablespoons crushed peanuts

DRESSING
3 tablespoons maple syrup
3 tablespoons lime juice
½ cup warm water
2 teaspoons rice vinegar
3 tablespoons fish sauce

Place the chicken in a large saucepan and cover with cold water. Cover with a cartouche and bring up to a near boil. Turn down the heat and gently simmer (water just moving slightly) for 10 minutes. Turn off the heat and leave the chicken to cool in the poaching liquid.

Whilst the chicken is poaching, make the dressing.

Place all the ingredients into a bowl and whisk to combine.

Shred the chicken and place in a large bowl. Add the vegetables, herbs and chilli to the chicken. Pour the dressing over the salad and gently toss to combine.

Place into four bowls and sprinkle each bowl with 1 tablespoon each of crushed peanuts.

NOTE: Barbequed chicken can also be used, if you are short on time.

Serves 4

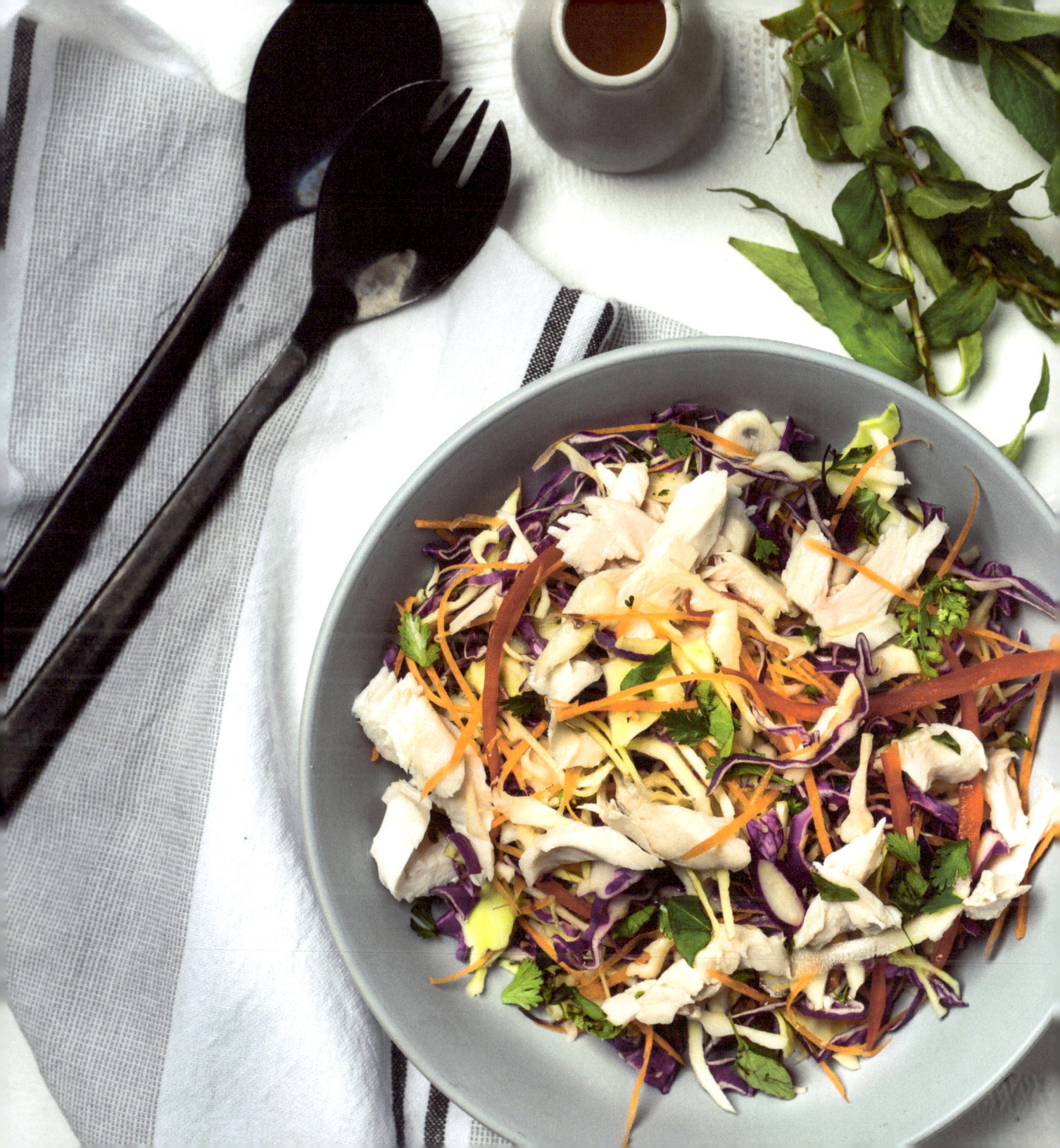

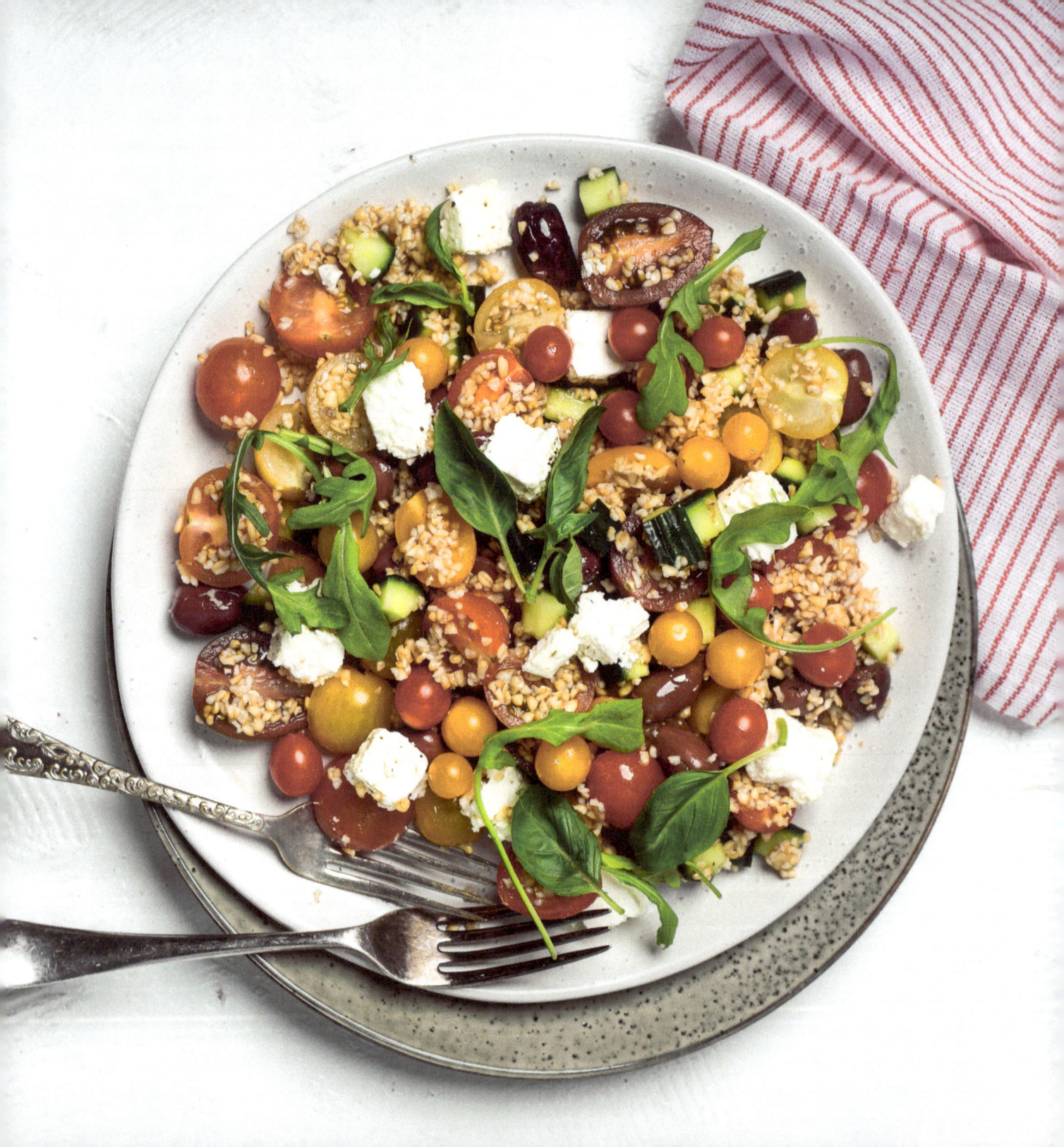

Mediterranean Salad

Bulgur wheat is a cereal grain made from pre-cooked cracked wheat. Bulgur wheat is a good source of fibre, manganese, magnesium and iron, and is quick to prepare.

200g Bulgur wheat

400g cherry tomatoes, cut in half

2 tablespoons kalamata olives, pitted

1 small cucumber, cut into cubes

Small bunch of basil leaves

200g feta cheese

DRESSING

3 tablespoons olive oil

2 tablespoons balsamic vinegar

Salt and pepper

Place the Bulgur wheat in a heatproof bowl and cover with boiling water for 10 minutes. Drain and place in a large bowl.

Combine dressing ingredients in a jar and shake to combine.

Add tomatoes, cucumber and olives to the Bulgur wheat, add dressing and mix thoroughly. Add basil and top with the feta cheese.

This salad can be eaten on its own or can be served on the side with lamb, chicken or haloumi cheese.

SERVES 2

The Main Event

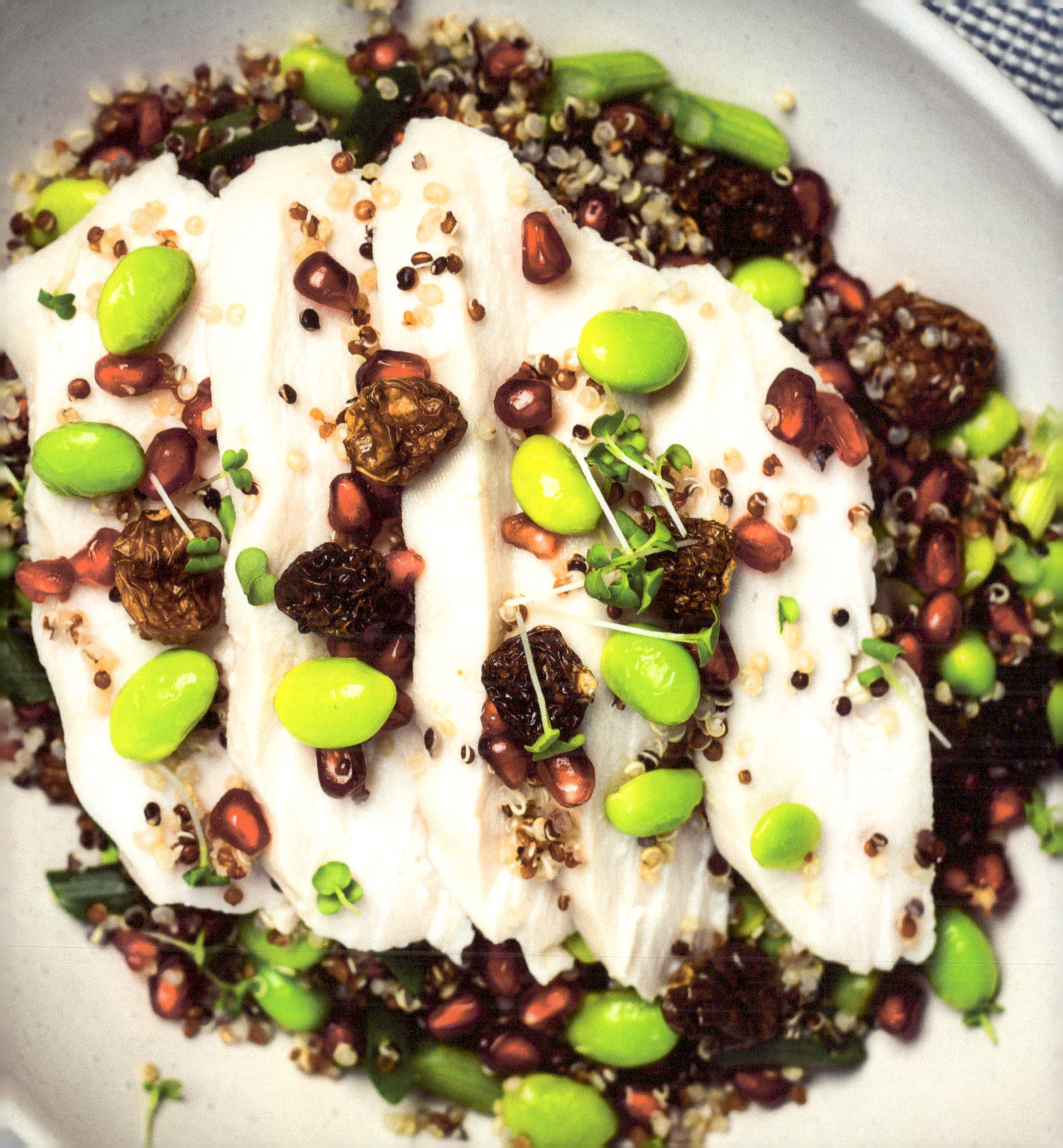

Black Bean Burrito Bowl

Black beans contain fibre, protein, carbohydrates, fat, folate, iron, magnesium, zinc, calcium and potassium. Canned black beans are convenient and add more protein and fibre to your diet whilst keeping it low in fat.

1 tablespoons light olive oil

1 red capsicum, cubed

1 yellow capsicum, cubed

1 red onion diced

1 garlic clove, minced

1 cup basmati rice, rinsed and drained

400ml of salsa

1 red chilli, sliced

40g packet of burrito spice mix (or 2 teaspoons ground cumin and 1 teaspoon chilli powder, ½ teaspoon salt)

375ml chicken stock

425g can black beans, drained, rinsed

425g can of corn, drained, rinsed

TO SERVE

1 avocado sliced

4 tablespoons pot set Greek Yoghurt

1 lime cut into quarters

Coriander, garnish

SERVES 4

Add 1 tablespoon of oil to the pressure cooker pot. Sauté onion, garlic and capsicum for approximately 1-2 minutes then add the spice and cook for 1-2 minutes or until aromatic. Add the drained rice to the pan and toast for a minute or two.

Add the salsa, chilli, stock and stir well.

Place lid on pressure cooker, lock it then bring the cooker to high pressure, over high heat. Reduce the heat to stabilise the pressure and cook for 5 minutes.

Release the pressure using the cold-water method and unlock the lid.

Add the drained beans and corn to the pot and heat through.

TO SERVE: divide between four bowls then add sliced avocado and 1 tablespoon of yoghurt into each bowl and a wedge of lime.

Garnish with coriander.

Combining beans and rice makes your meal a complete protein.

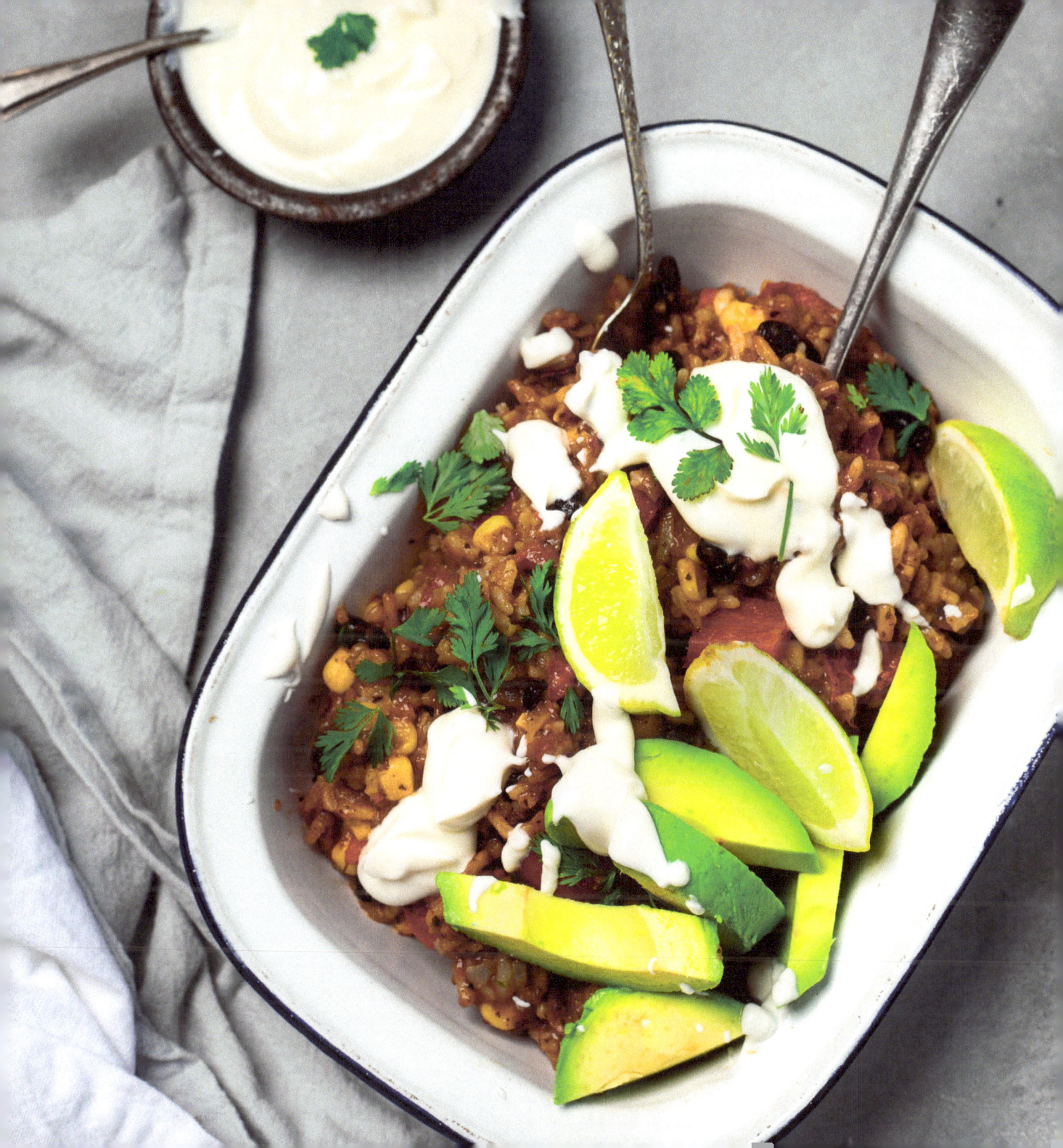

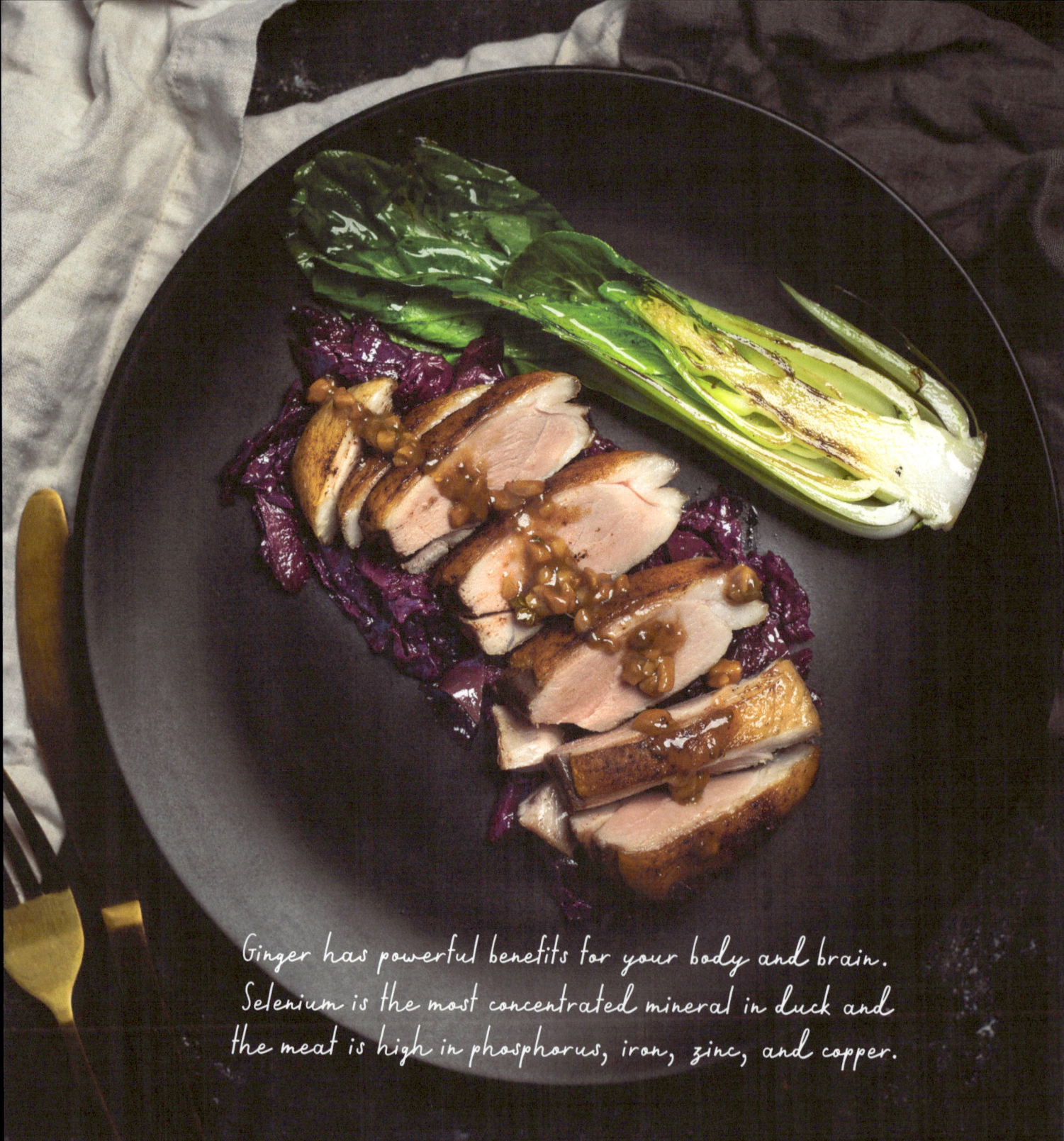

Ginger has powerful benefits for your body and brain. Selenium is the most concentrated mineral in duck and the meat is high in phosphorus, iron, zinc, and copper.

Duck Breast with Ginger and Thyme Sauce

4 duck breasts

2 cm piece of fresh ginger, grated

50g chopped mixed nuts

2 teaspoons chopped thyme

3 tablespoons nut oil

1 tablespoon dark brown sugar

3 tablespoons orange juice

3 tablespoons marsala

2 tablespoons balsamic vinegar

300ml chicken stock

1 teaspoon chia seeds to thicken or 1 tablespoon of arrowroot

Preheat oven to 180° Celsius.

Pat dry the duck breasts with paper towel.

Score the duck skin with a sharp knife, being careful not to cut the flesh.

Season the duck with sea salt and black pepper.

Starting with a cold heavy pan, place the duck breasts skin side down over medium heat. Cook for 7 minutes. Turn breasts over and sear the other side for 2 minutes.

Transfer the pan to the oven and roast for approximately 10 minutes for medium to well done, depending on the thickness of the breast.

Rest the duck for 10 minutes prior to serving.

SAUCE

Heat the oil in a frying pan over a low to medium heat and add the grated fresh ginger, nuts, thyme and sugar. Cook for 1 minute, then add the orange juice, marsala, balsamic vinegar and stock and simmer for approximately 4 minutes.

Add the chia seeds or 1 tablespoon of arrowroot mixed with 1 tablespoon of water and continue to simmer, stirring to thicken to a light syrupy consistency.

Serve the duck and sauce with red cabbage and bok choy.

SERVES 4

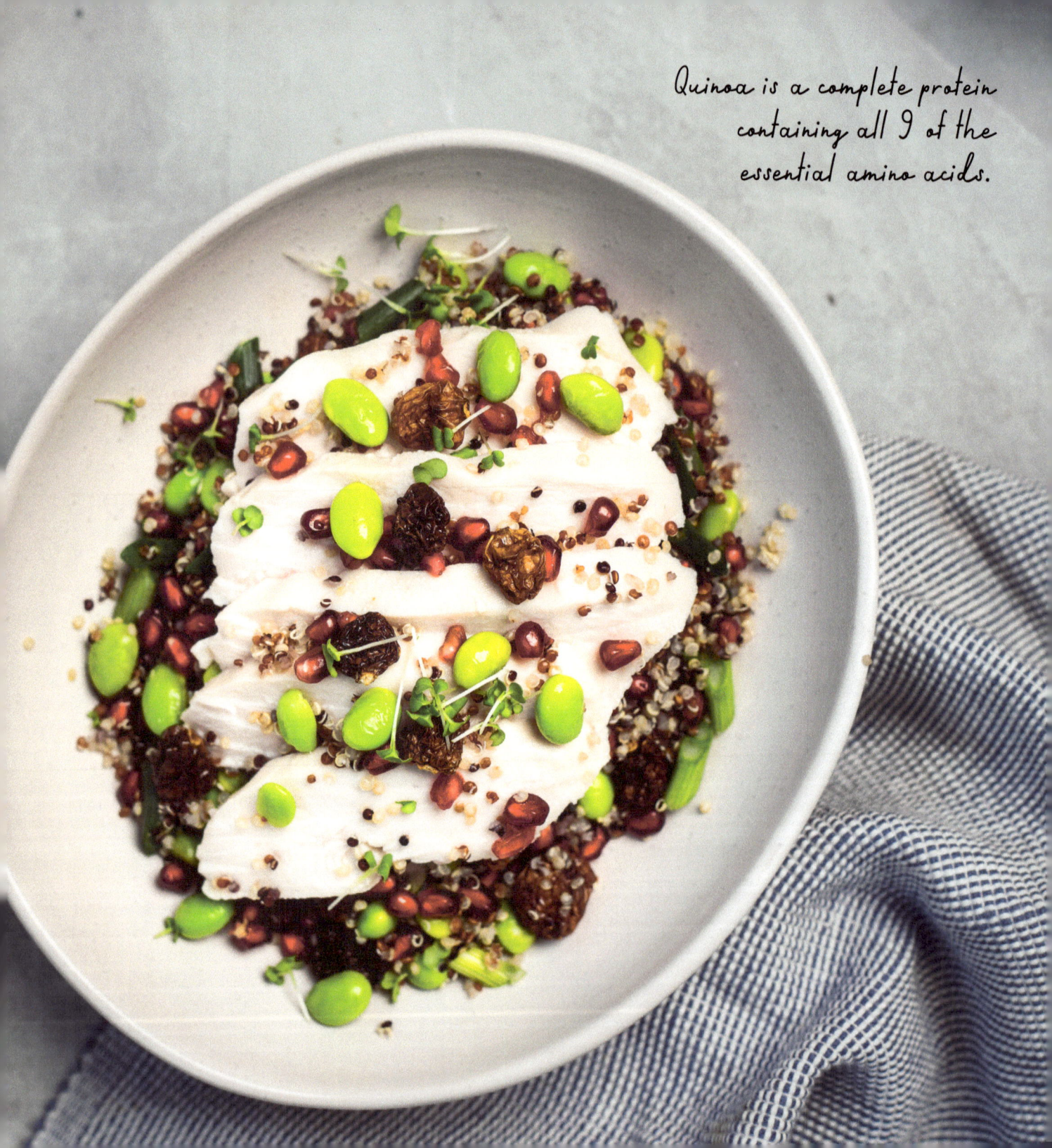

Quinoa is a complete protein containing all 9 of the essential amino acids.

Poached Chicken on Jewelled Quinoa Salad

4 chicken breasts

DRESSING
1 tablespoon of lemon juice
1 tablespoon of orange juice
80ml olive oil
Sea salt and ground black pepper

JEWELLED QUINOA
200g quinoa
1 bunch dill chopped
2 spring onions, thinly sliced
40g goldenberry
1 pomegranate arils
100g edamame beans
Salt and pepper
Micro herbs, garnish

Blanch the edamame beans in a pan of boiling water for 2-3 minutes. Drain and cool

Place the chicken in a large saucepan and cover with cold water. Cover with a cartouche and bring up to a near boil. Turn down the heat and gently simmer (water just moving slightly) for 10 minutes. Turn off the heat and leave the chicken to cool in the poaching liquid.

Whilst the chicken is poaching, make the dressing.

Place all the ingredients into a bowl and whisk to combine. Season with salt and pepper.

When the chicken is cool enough to handle, slice the chicken. Toss in some of the dressing to coat generously.

Boil the quinoa in the poaching liquid until tender. Approximately 10 minutes.

Whilst the quinoa is cooking, place the spring onions, goldenberry, dill, pomegranate arils, and edamame beans into a bowl.

When the quinoa is cooked, drain and then add to the bowl with some of the reserved dressing. Season to taste.

To serve: divide the quinoa between four plates, topping with some sliced poached chicken.

Garnish with micro herbs. Serve immediately.

SERVES 4

Prawn, Cannellini Bean and Quinoa Salad

Quinoa is gluten free, high in protein, fibre and minerals.

20 cooked and peeled prawns
60ml olive oil
60ml lemon juice
200g quinoa
400g can of cannellini beans, drained and rinsed
1 preserved lemon quarter, white pith removed, rind finely chopped
250g of cherry tomatoes, cut in half
½ bunch of mint, picked and roughly chopped

DRESSING
30ml lemon juice
90ml olive oil
Sea salt and ground black pepper

Combine oil and lemon juice in a bowl and season with salt and pepper. Add the prawns and toss to combine, then cover and chill until required.

Place the washed quinoa in a medium pot with 1 ½ cups of water. Bring to the boil then lower the heat and simmer, uncovered until the quinoa is tender, about 10 minutes.

For the dressing, whisk the olive oil, lemon juice and mustard until combined. Season with salt and pepper.

In a large bowl gently combine beans, tomatoes, preserved lemon and herbs. Add in the quinoa and stir through. Pour over the dressing and mix well.

Transfer the salad to a serving platter. Drain the prawns, discarding the marinade and arrange prawns on top.

Garnish with extra mint. Serve immediately.

SERVES 4

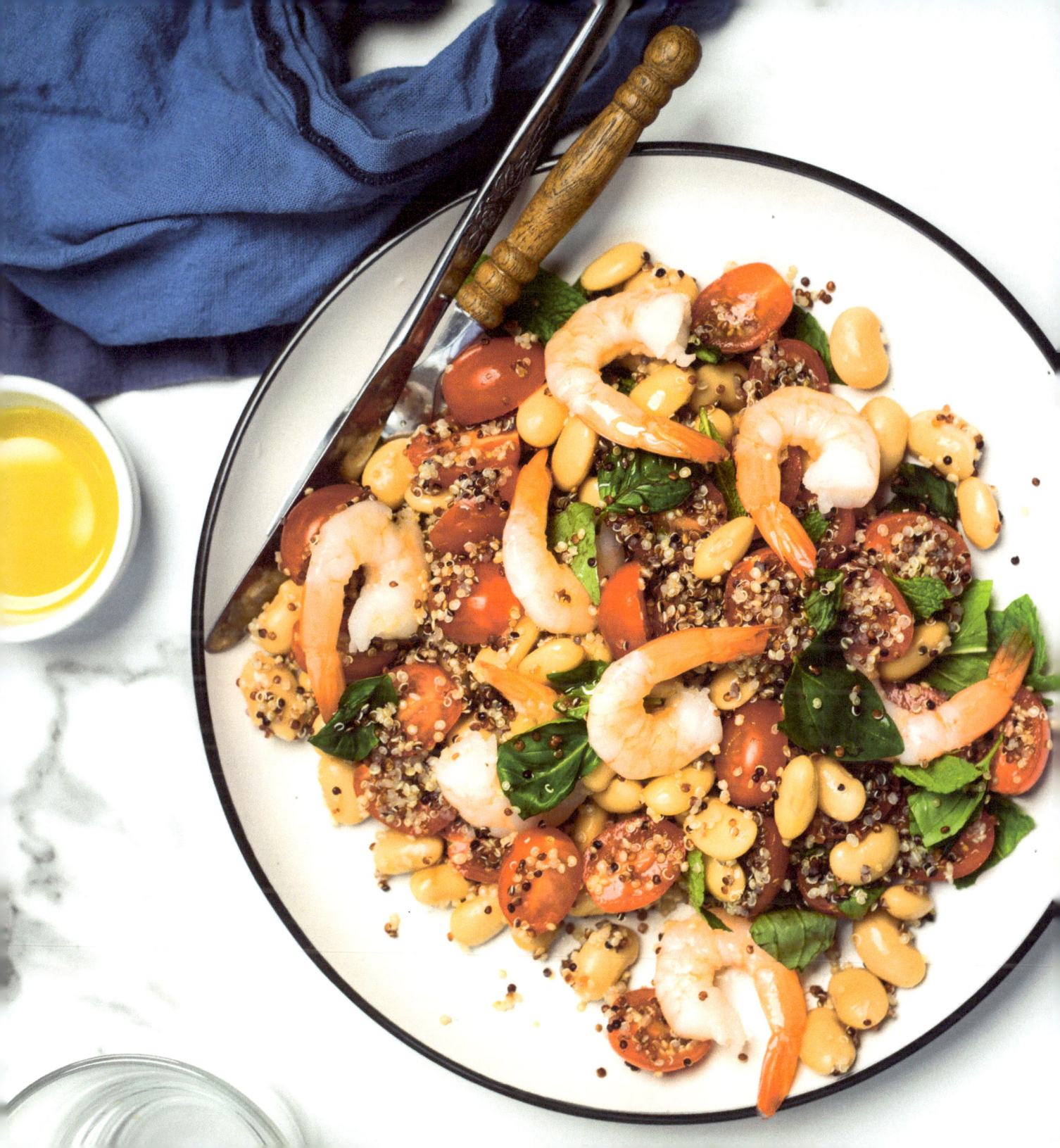

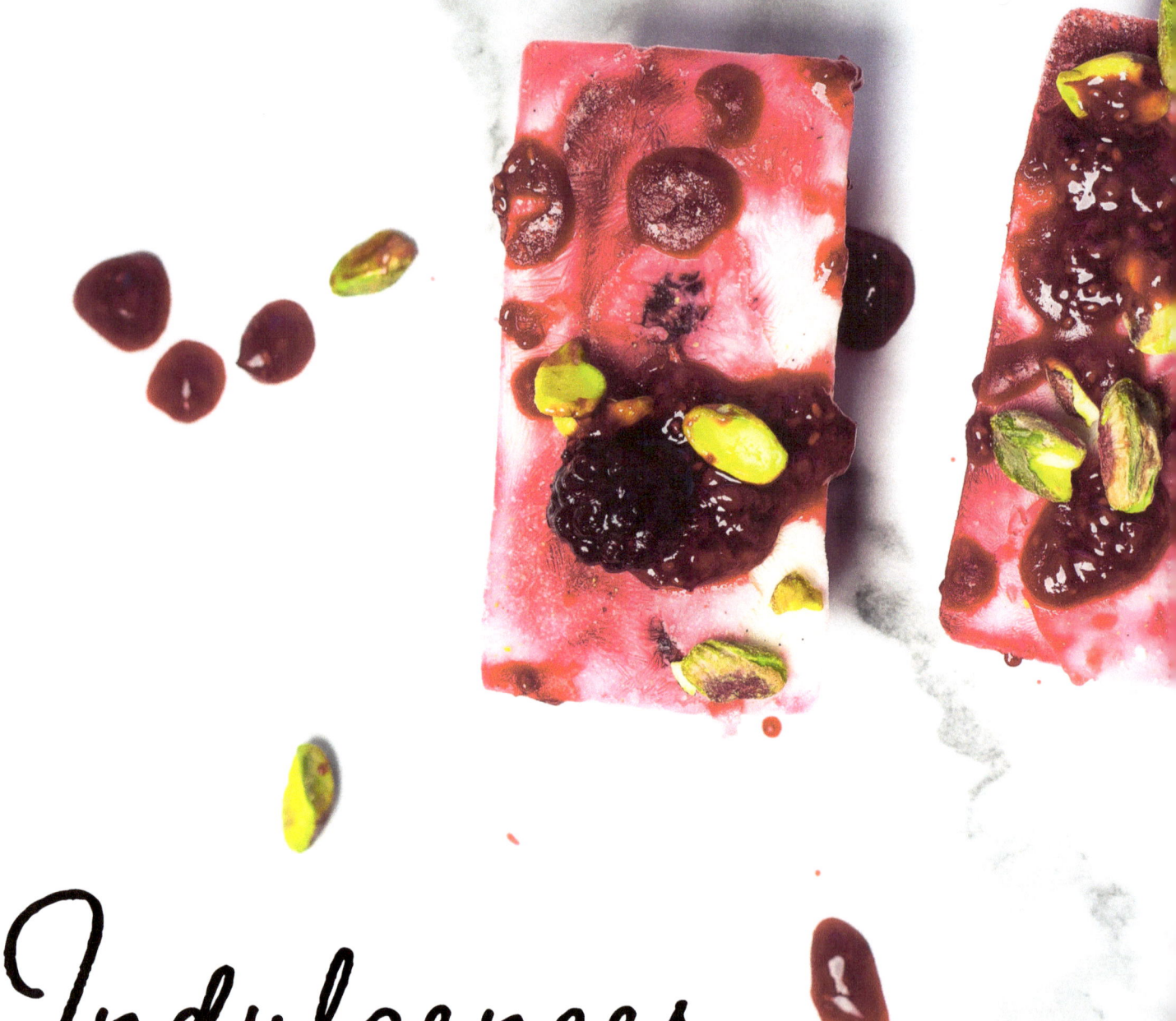

Indulgences

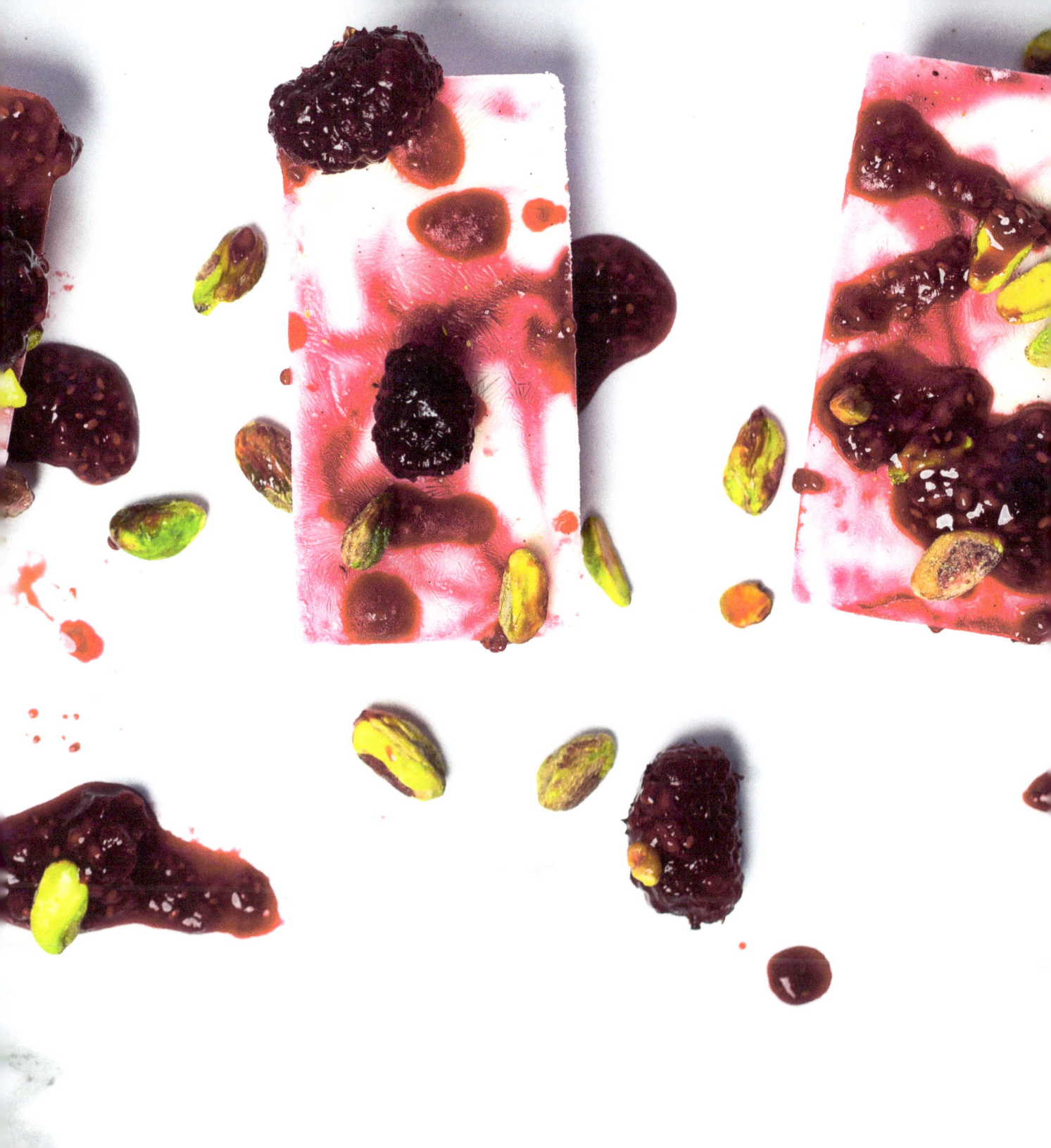

Vegan Blueberry Ice Cream

Blueberries are loaded with nutrients, vitamins, fibre, antioxidants, phytochemicals and flavonoids.

2 ripe bananas, sliced and frozen

2 cups frozen blueberries or berries of choice

Place frozen banana slices and frozen berries in a food processor and pulse until the fruit starts to break up. Scrape down the sides of the bowl and then blend on high until smooth. This may take a little time, 2-3 minutes, but persevere.

Scoop into bowls and serve immediately or alternatively scoop into a glass and top with berries, nuts, coconut shards.

NOTE: Best eaten at time of making however you can freeze the ice cream. Remove from freezer 10 minutes prior to eating to soften a little.

SERVES 4

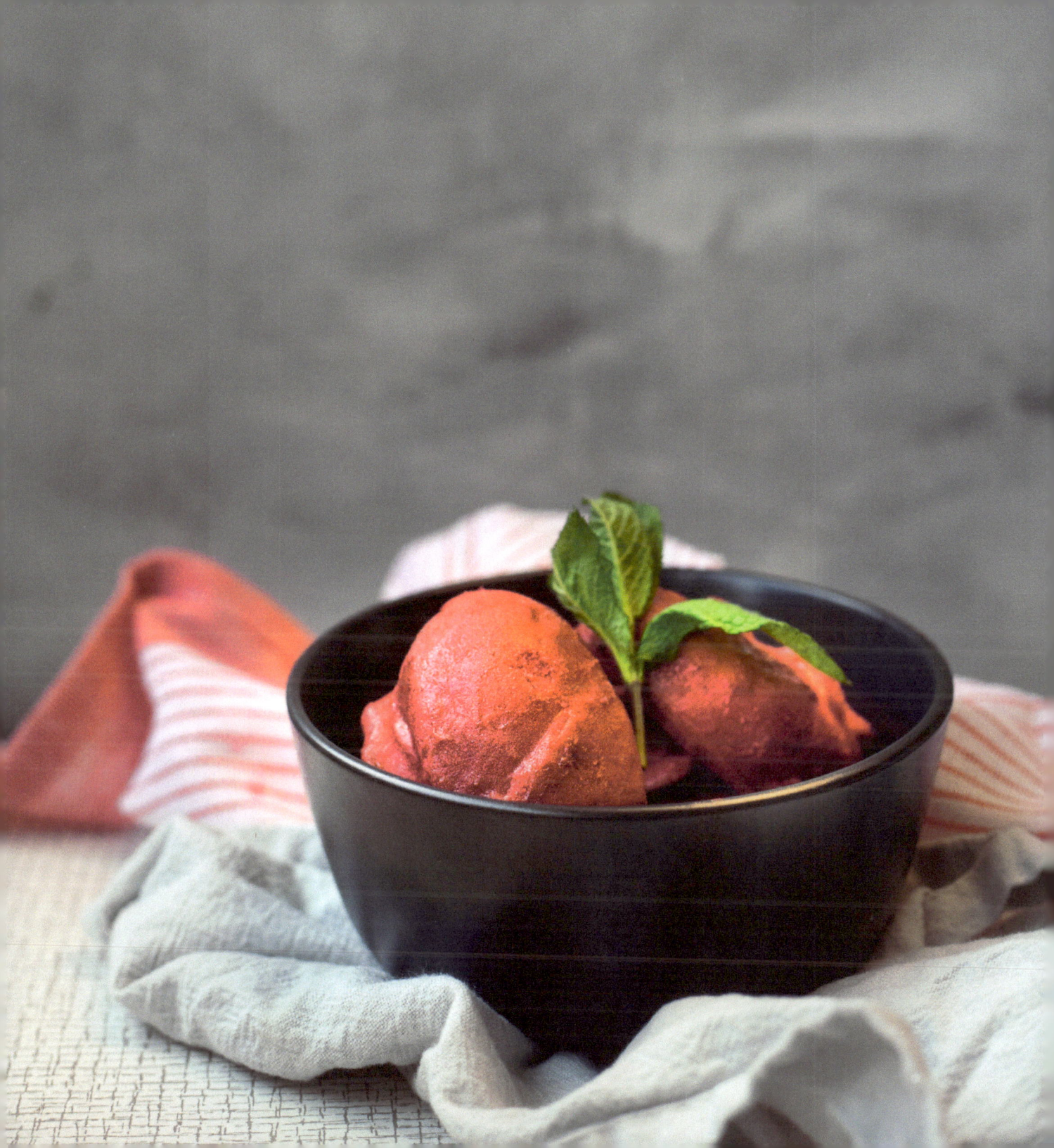

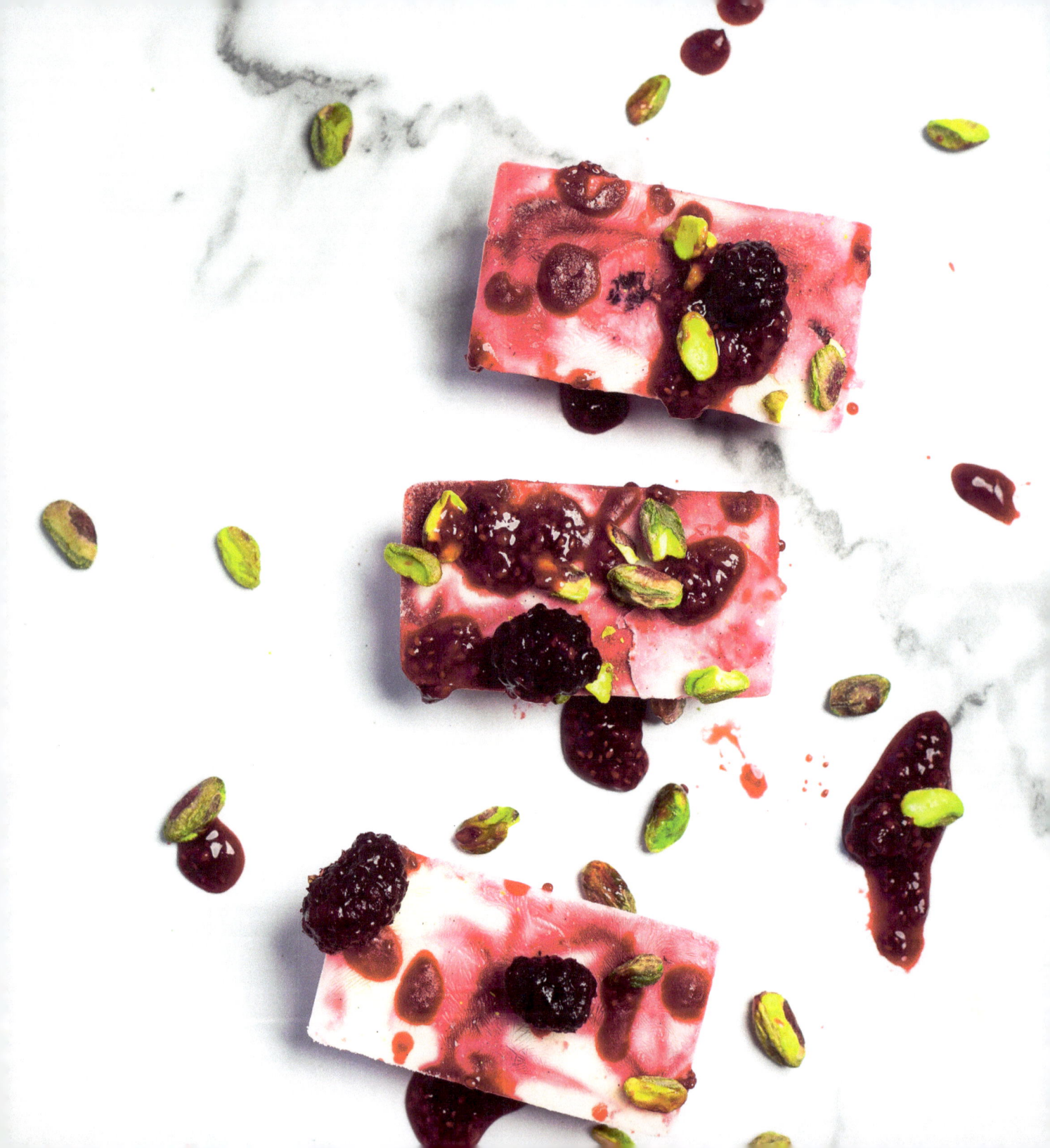

Berry Frozen Yoghurt Bars

3 cups frozen mulberries or berries of your choice
125ml maple syrup
1 tablespoon vanilla bean paste
3 cups Greek yoghurt

EQUIPMENT
Silicone muffin mould

Place berries in a pot and heat over medium heat for approximately 5 minutes or until just starting to soften and bleed.

Combine yoghurt, maple syrup and vanilla bean paste in a bowl and stir to combine.

Pour half the mixture into each hole. Add half the berries and swirl through. Pour over remaining yoghurt and swirl with some juice.

Freeze overnight.

Stand at room temperature for 10 minutes then unmold.

Serve topped with some berries and juice.

NOTE: For a healthy treat for children, mix all ingredients together and spoon into popsicle molds then freeze overnight.

Mulberries contain high amounts of iron and vitamin C as well as vitamins E and K and potassium.

SERVES 10

Avocado Brownies

250g avocado
150g dark chocolate
60ml coconut oil
60g pitted dates, chopped
½ teaspoon salt
3 eggs, whisked
½ teaspoon baking powder
80g almond meal
1 teaspoon honey
Crushed pistachio nuts for garnish – optional

Preheat oven to 170° Celsius.

Line a 20cm square baking tin with parchment paper.

Finely mash the avocado.

Place the chocolate and coconut oil in a heatproof bowl. Stand the bowl over a pan of gently simmering water to melt the chocolate, stirring occasionally.

Stir the mashed avocado into the chocolate.

Add the chopped dates and salt to this bowl, using a stick blender, pulse the chocolate mixture until smooth.

Add the eggs and baking powder, pulse again until smooth then add the almond meal and honey. Combine with a silicone spatula.

Transfer the mixture into the prepared tin and bake in the middle of the oven for 25-30 minutes. Insert a skewer into the brownies and if it comes out clean the brownies are ready. Allow to cool in the tin and then transfer to a wire rack to cool completely before cutting.

Top with crushed pistachio nuts.

Serves 4

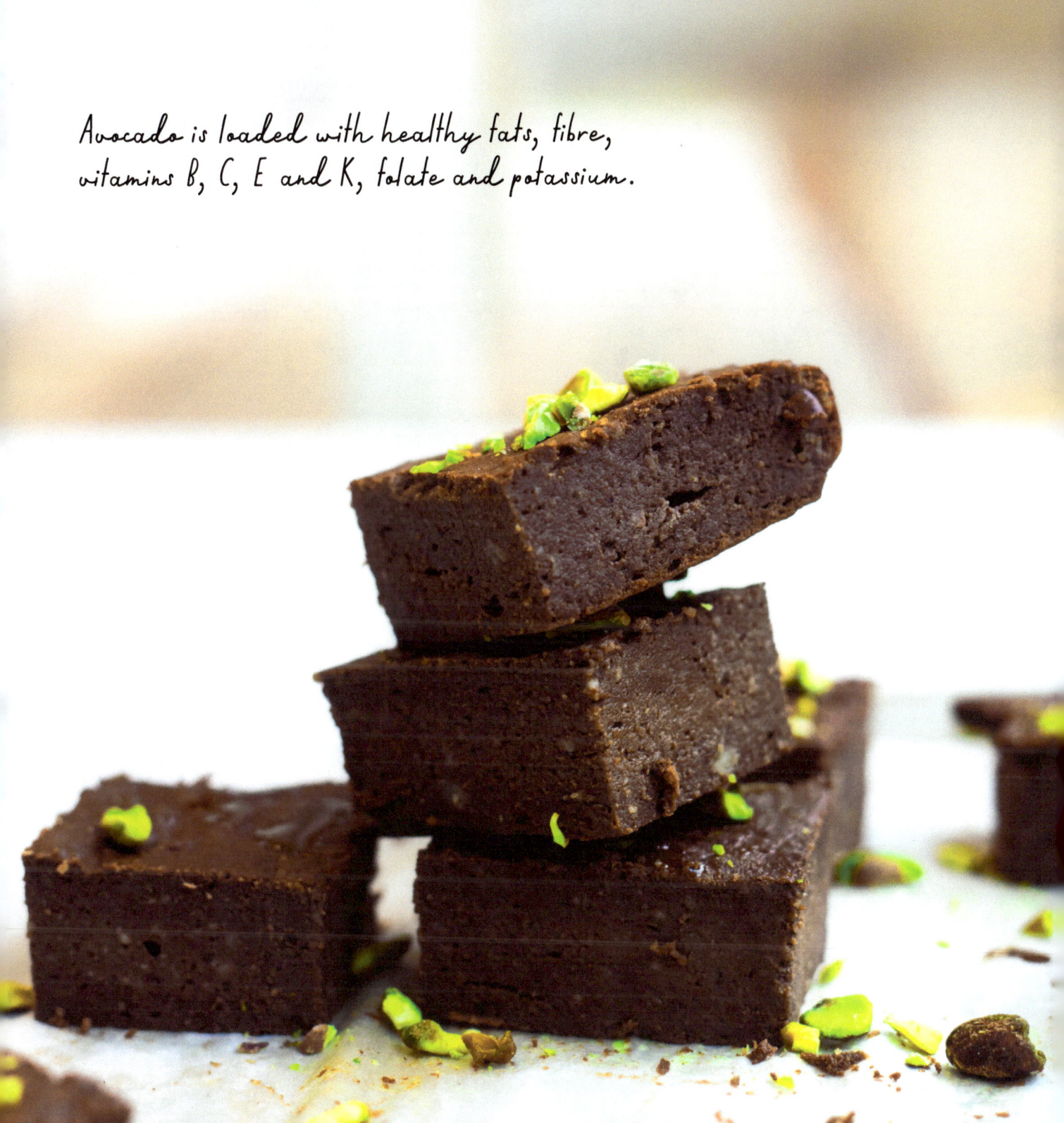

Avocado is loaded with healthy fats, fibre, vitamins B, C, E and K, folate and potassium.

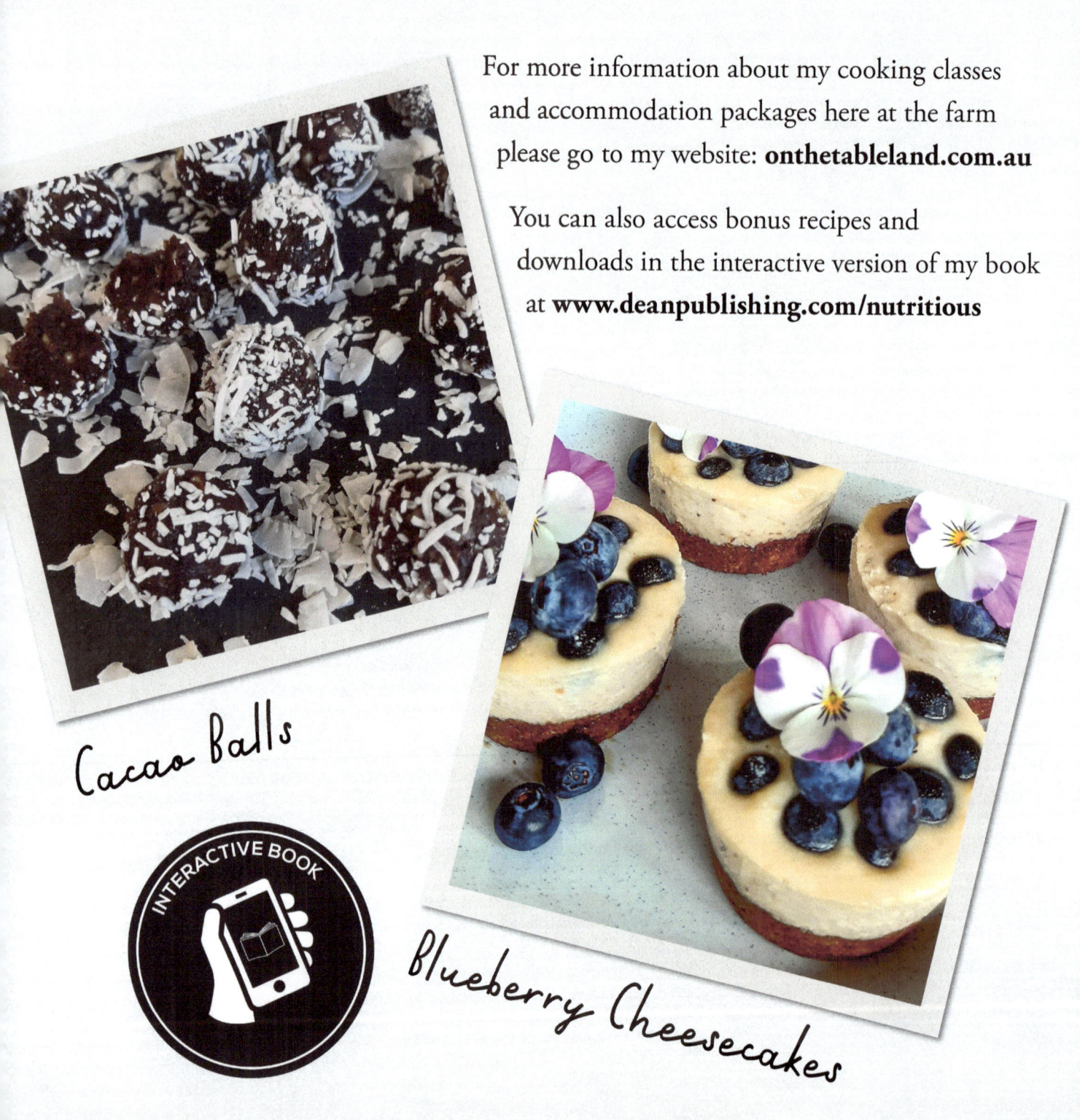

For more information about my cooking classes and accommodation packages here at the farm please go to my website: **onthetableland.com.au**

You can also access bonus recipes and downloads in the interactive version of my book at **www.deanpublishing.com/nutritious**

Cacao Balls

Blueberry Cheesecakes

www.ingramcontent.com/pod-product-compliance
Lightning Source LLC
Chambersburg PA
CBHW041459220426
43661CB00016B/1200